THE ILEOSTOMY DIET COOKBOOK FOR NEWLY DIAGNOSED 2024.

Including 6-Week Ileostomy Recovery Plan, Delicious Low-Fiber Recipes for beginners, Meal Ideas & Prep Tips to Promote Smooth Healing.

DR. RAYMOND JOHNSON.

Copyright © 2024 by Dr. Raymond Johnson

All rights reserved. No part of this publication may be reproduced, distributed, or transmitted in any form or by any means, including photocopying, recording, or other electronic or mechanical methods, without the prior written permission of the publisher, except in the case of brief quotations embodied in critical reviews and certain other noncommercial uses permitted by copyright law.

CONTENTS

INTRODUCTION 5

CHAPTER 1: UNDERSTANDING ILEOSTOMY 7

    What Is an Ileostomy? 7

    Why Do You Need a Special Diet After Ileostomy Surgery? 10

    How Does Diet Affect Ileostomy Recovery? 11

    The Importance of a Well-Planned Diet 13

CHAPTER 2: YOUR 6-WEEK ILEOSTOMY RECOVERY PLAN 16

    Week 1: Introduction to Soft Foods 16

    Week 2: Gradual Introduction of Low-Fiber Foods ... 18

    Week 3: Incorporating Balanced Nutrients 20

    Week 4: Exploring Flavorful Options 23

    Week 5: Enhancing Variety and Texture 25

    Week 6: Sustainable Diet for Long-Term Healing 28

Chapter 3: Essential Tips for Cooking and Meal Preparation 31

    Kitchen Essentials for Ileostomy Patients 31

    Smart Meal Planning Strategies 34

    Safe Cooking Techniques for Easy Digestion 38

Stocking Your Pantry with Ileostomy-Friendly
Ingredients 44

Chapter 4: Breakfast Recipes for a Nourishing Start 51

   10 Energizing Smoothies and Shakes 51

   10 Soft and Easily Digestible Breakfast Bowls 56

   10 Creative Egg Dishes and Alternatives 63

   10 Quick Grab-and-Go Options 73

Chapter 5: Lunch Ideas for Sustained Energy 81

   10 Wholesome Soups and Broths 81

   10 Protein-Packed Salads and Wraps 91

   10 Nutrient-Dense Sandwiches and Toasts 99

   10 Portable Lunchbox Favorites 106

Chapter 6: Dinner Recipes for Comfort and Healing ... 116

   Nourishing One-Pot Meals 116

   Flavorful Pasta and Rice Dishes 122

   Tender Meat and Fish Entrées 135

   Veggie-Centric Options for Plant-Based Delights ... 146

Chapter 7: Snacks and Sides to Support Your Diet 160

   Crunchy and Chewy Snack Ideas 160

   Satisfying Side Dishes for Every Meal 164

   Homemade Dips and Spreads 167

   Nutrient-Rich Trail Mixes and Bars 169

Chapter 8: Desserts for Sweet Indulgences 171

Soft and Decadent Puddings 171
Fruity Sorbets and Gelatin Treats............................174
Baked Goods Made Easy on the Digestive System .176
Guilt-Free Dessert Alternatives................................178
Conclusion...181

INTRODUCTION

Welcome to The Ileostomy Diet Cookbook for Newly diagnosed, your comprehensive guide to navigating the world of nutrition post-ileostomy surgery.

Whether you're a recent ileostomy patient or supporting a loved one through their recovery journey, this book is designed to empower you with the knowledge and tools needed to thrive.

An ileostomy, though life-changing, doesn't have to hinder your enjoyment of food or compromise your nutritional needs. With the right guidance and understanding, you can embark on a fulfilling culinary journey that supports your healing process and enhances your overall well-being.

In these pages, you'll find a wealth of information curated by myself, Dr. Raymond Johnson. Drawing upon years of experience in gastroenterology and nutrition, I'm bringing to you, a comprehensive six-week recovery plan, delicious low-fiber recipes, meal ideas, and practical preparation tips.

While an ileostomy undoubtedly presents its challenges, it also opens the door to a new chapter of life—one filled with resilience, adaptability, and yes, even culinary exploration. However, adjusting to life with an ileostomy requires patience, education, and a supportive community. That's where this book comes in.

Throughout the following chapters, we'll delve into essential topics such as understanding your digestive system post-surgery, mastering portion control, managing potential dietary restrictions, and creating a balanced meal plan tailored to your unique needs. Additionally, we'll explore the importance of hydration, supplementation, and mindful eating practices to optimize your recovery and promote long-term health.

But this book isn't just about information—it's about transformation. So, dear reader, whether you're embarking on your own journey towards healing or extending a helping hand to someone in need, I invite you to join me on this culinary adventure. Together, we'll debunk myths, overcome obstacles, and celebrate the beauty of resilience in the face of adversity.

CHAPTER 1: UNDERSTANDING ILEOSTOMY

Embarking on the journey of recovery after ileostomy surgery can feel like stepping into the unknown. From adjusting to life with a stoma to navigating dietary changes, there are numerous aspects to consider as you embark on this new chapter of your life. In this chapter, we will delve into the fundamentals of understanding ileostomy, exploring what it entails, why a special diet is necessary post-surgery, and how your dietary choices can impact your recovery journey. Additionally, we'll emphasize the importance of a well-planned diet tailored to your individual needs, setting the stage for a smoother, more nourishing path toward healing and vitality.

What Is an Ileostomy?

An ileostomy is a surgical procedure that involves creating an opening in the abdomen, known as a stoma, to reroute the flow of digestive waste from the small intestine directly to the surface of the abdomen. This procedure is typically performed when a portion of the colon or rectum is removed or bypassed due to medical conditions such as inflammatory bowel disease (Crohn's disease or ulcerative colitis), colorectal cancer, diverticulitis, or other digestive disorders.

The stoma, which resembles a small, pinkish protrusion on the abdomen, is formed by bringing a portion of the small intestine (ileum) through an incision in the abdominal wall. Waste products, including stool and digestive fluids, exit the body through the stoma and are collected in a pouching system attached to the skin around the stoma.

There are different types of ileostomies, including:

1. **End ileostomy:** In this type of ileostomy, the entire colon and rectum are removed, and the end of the ileum is brought through the abdominal wall to create the stoma.

2. **Loop ileostomy:** In a loop ileostomy, a loop of the ileum is brought to the surface of the abdomen to form the stoma. This type of ileostomy is often temporary and may be created to divert stool away from a diseased or injured portion of the intestine while it heals.

3. **Continent ileostomy:** Also known as a Kock pouch or continent ileostomy, this procedure involves creating a reservoir inside the abdomen

using a portion of the small intestine. A valve mechanism is constructed to control the flow of waste, allowing the patient to manage elimination by inserting a catheter into the pouch.

An ileostomy is a life-changing procedure that can have a significant impact on a person's physical, emotional, and social well-being. While it may require adjustments and adaptation, many individuals with ileostomies lead active and fulfilling lives, participating in various activities, including work, exercise, and travel.

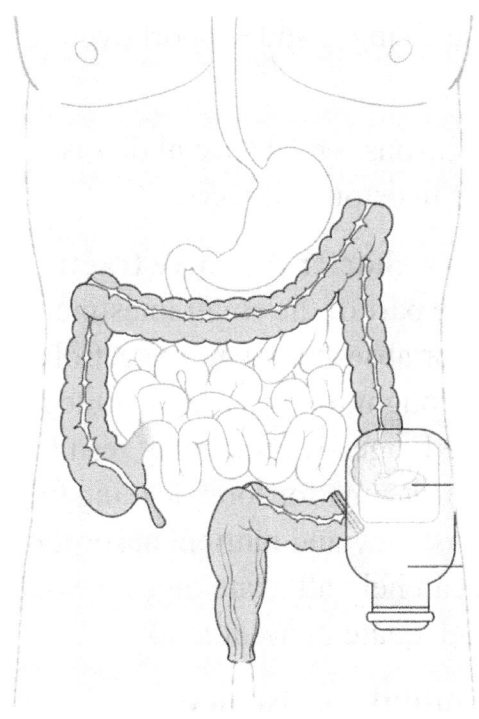

Why Do You Need a Special Diet After Ileostomy Surgery?

After undergoing ileostomy surgery, it's crucial to adopt a special diet to promote healing, prevent complications, and ensure optimal digestion and nutrition. The surgery alters the digestive process by bypassing or removing a portion of the intestines, which can impact how nutrients are absorbed and how the body processes food. Therefore, dietary modifications are necessary to accommodate these changes and support overall health and well-being.

There are several reasons why a special diet is recommended after ileostomy surgery:

1. **Adjusting to a shorter digestive tract:** In an ileostomy, the part of the small intestine that is responsible for absorbing water, electrolytes, and nutrients is brought to the surface of the abdomen. This shortened digestive tract may result in increased transit time for food, leading to changes in stool consistency and nutrient absorption. A special diet can help alleviate digestive discomfort and ensure adequate nutrient intake.

2. **Managing output consistency**

3. **Preventing blockages or obstructions**
4. **Minimizing gas production**
5. **Optimizing nutrient absorption**

How Does Diet Affect Ileostomy Recovery?

Understanding how diet affects ileostomy recovery is crucial for navigating the post-surgery journey with confidence and resilience. Your dietary choices play a significant role in shaping your recovery process, influencing everything from your energy levels and digestive comfort to the healing of your surgical site. Think of your diet as the fuel that powers your body's recovery engine—a well-balanced and nourishing diet can turbocharge your healing process, while poor dietary choices may throw a wrench in the works.

First and foremost, your diet directly impacts the output and consistency of stool from your stoma. Certain foods can either speed up or slow down digestion, affecting the frequency and texture of your bowel movements. By selecting foods that are gentle on your digestive system and easily digestible, you can help regulate stool consistency and minimize issues like diarrhea or constipation, which can disrupt your daily routine and compromise your comfort.

Moreover, your dietary intake directly influences your body's ability to heal and repair tissues post-surgery. Opting for nutrient-rich foods that are packed with vitamins, minerals, and antioxidants provides your body with the building blocks it needs to mend wounds, strengthen tissues, and fight off infections. Conversely, a diet lacking in essential nutrients can hinder the healing process and prolong recovery time, leaving you feeling fatigued, sluggish, and susceptible to complications.

Additionally, your diet plays a vital role in managing inflammation and promoting gut health—a critical aspect of ileostomy recovery. Certain foods, such as those rich in omega-3 fatty acids, anti-inflammatory spices, and probiotics, can help reduce inflammation in the body and support a healthy balance of gut bacteria. By incorporating these foods into your diet, you can soothe inflammation, promote tissue healing, and enhance overall well-being.

Furthermore, your dietary choices can impact your mood, energy levels, and overall quality of life during the recovery period. Opting for balanced meals and snacks that provide sustained energy throughout the day can help combat fatigue and keep you feeling alert, focused, and motivated. On the other hand, consuming highly processed foods, sugary snacks, or caffeine in excess may lead to energy crashes, mood swings, and decreased resilience to stress.

The Importance of a Well-Planned Diet

Navigating life with an ileostomy requires more than just a casual approach to eating—it calls for a strategic and thoughtful approach to nourishment. A well-planned diet isn't just a luxury—it's a necessity for promoting optimal health, supporting recovery, and enhancing overall well-being. Here's why:

Firstly, a well-planned diet ensures that you're getting all the essential nutrients your body needs to thrive. Following ileostomy surgery, your digestive system undergoes significant changes that can affect nutrient absorption and utilization. By carefully selecting a variety of nutrient-dense foods, including fruits, vegetables, lean proteins, whole grains, and healthy fats, you can ensure that your body receives the vitamins, minerals, and antioxidants it needs to function optimally and support the healing process.

Moreover, a well-planned diet plays a crucial role in managing digestive symptoms and promoting gastrointestinal health. Certain foods can either exacerbate or alleviate common issues such as diarrhea, gas, bloating, and abdominal discomfort. By identifying trigger foods and incorporating gut-friendly options into your diet, you can minimize discomfort, improve stool consistency, and enhance overall digestive comfort.

Furthermore, a well-planned diet helps stabilize blood sugar levels and sustain energy levels throughout the day. Choosing balanced meals and snacks that combine complex carbohydrates, lean proteins, and healthy fats provides a steady source of fuel for your body, preventing energy crashes and mood swings. This is particularly important during the recovery period when your body requires extra energy and nutrients to support healing and repair.

Additionally, a well-planned diet promotes long-term health and reduces the risk of complications associated with ileostomy surgery. By prioritizing whole, minimally processed foods and limiting intake of highly processed, sugary, and fatty foods, you can support cardiovascular health, maintain a healthy weight, and reduce the risk of chronic diseases such as diabetes, heart disease, and certain cancers.

Furthermore, a well-planned diet fosters a positive relationship with food and promotes a sense of empowerment and control over your health. By taking an active role in planning and preparing meals, you can explore new foods, flavors, and culinary techniques, expanding your palate and enhancing your enjoyment of eating. This sense of agency can boost confidence, reduce anxiety, and foster a greater sense of well-being as you navigate life with an ileostomy.

CHAPTER 2: YOUR 6-WEEK ILEOSTOMY RECOVERY PLAN

Embarking on the road to recovery after ileostomy surgery requires patience, perseverance, and a well-thought-out plan. In this chapter, we will outline a comprehensive six-week recovery plan designed to support your healing journey, nourish your body, and empower you with the tools and knowledge needed to thrive post-surgery.

Each week of the recovery plan focuses on specific dietary goals and milestones, gradually introducing new foods, flavors, and textures while prioritizing digestive comfort, nutrient intake, and overall well-being.

Week 1: Introduction to Soft Foods

Welcome to Week 1 of your ileostomy recovery journey! In this pivotal first week, our focus is on gentle nourishment and easing your digestive system into the post-surgery phase. We'll be introducing soft, easily digestible foods that provide essential nutrients while minimizing discomfort and promoting healing.

After ileostomy surgery, your digestive system may need some time to adjust to its new normal.

Soft foods are gentle on the digestive tract, making them an ideal choice for this transitional period. They're easy to chew, swallow, and digest, reducing the strain on your gastrointestinal system and promoting optimal nutrient absorption.

Throughout Week 1, aim to incorporate a variety of soft foods into your meals and snacks, including:

1. **Cooked vegetables**: Steamed or boiled vegetables such as carrots, squash, zucchini, and potatoes are easy to digest and provide essential vitamins and minerals.

2. **Ripe fruits**: Opt for soft, ripe fruits like bananas, avocados, melons, and cooked applesauce. These fruits are gentle on the stomach and rich in fiber, vitamins, and antioxidants.

3. **Cooked grains:** Choose soft, well-cooked grains such as rice, oatmeal, and quinoa. These grains provide a good source of carbohydrates and fiber, promoting digestive regularity and satiety.

4. **Lean proteins**: Incorporate lean, tender proteins like chicken, fish, tofu, and eggs into your meals. These protein sources are easy to digest and provide essential amino acids for tissue repair and muscle maintenance.

5. **Dairy alternatives:** If you tolerate dairy well, opt for soft dairy products like yogurt, cottage cheese, and soft cheeses. Alternatively, explore non-dairy options such as almond milk, soy yogurt, and dairy-free cheese substitutes.

Remember to chew your food thoroughly and eat slowly to aid digestion and prevent discomfort.

Stay hydrated by sipping water throughout the day, aiming for at least 8-10 cups of fluid intake daily.

As you navigate Week 1, listen to your body and pay attention to how different foods make you feel. Keep a food diary to track your symptoms and identify any potential trigger foods or intolerances. And most importantly, be gentle with yourself as you adjust to this new chapter of your journey.

Week 2: Gradual Introduction of Low-Fiber Foods.

Welcome to Week 2 of your ileostomy recovery journey! This week, we'll continue building upon the foundation established in Week 1 by gradually introducing low-fiber foods into your diet. Low-fiber foods are easier to digest and less likely to cause discomfort or irritation to your digestive system, making them an excellent choice as you transition toward a more varied diet.

As you incorporate low-fiber foods into your meals and snacks, keep the following guidelines in mind:

1. **Choose refined grains:** Opt for refined grains such as white bread, white rice, and pasta instead of their whole grain counterparts. These foods are lower in fiber and less likely to cause bowel obstruction or irritation to your stoma.

2. **Include lean proteins:** Continue to include lean sources of protein in your diet, such as poultry, fish, tofu, and eggs. These proteins are gentle on the digestive system and provide essential nutrients for healing and recovery.

3. **Experiment with cooked vegetables:** Expand your repertoire of cooked vegetables by incorporating low-fiber options such as peeled and cooked carrots, green beans, and well-cooked spinach. Avoid raw vegetables or those with tough skins or seeds, as they may be harder to digest.

4. **Explore canned fruits:** Canned fruits, especially those packed in their own juices or light syrup, can be a convenient and easy-to-digest option. Choose fruits like peaches, pears, and pineapple, and avoid varieties with added sugars or high fiber content.

5. **Include dairy in moderation:** If you tolerate dairy well, continue to include soft dairy products like yogurt and cottage cheese in your diet.

However, be mindful of lactose intolerance or dairy sensitivities, and opt for lactose-free or dairy-free alternatives if needed.

6. **Incorporate nut butters and seedless spreads:** Spreadable options like smooth nut butters (e.g., peanut butter, almond butter) and seedless jams or jellies can add flavor and nutrition to your meals without the added fiber from whole nuts or seeds.

Throughout Week 2, pay attention to how your body responds to the introduction of new foods and adjust your diet accordingly. Stay hydrated by drinking plenty of water and other fluids, and continue to chew your food thoroughly to aid digestion.

By gradually introducing low-fiber foods into your diet this week, you're taking another important step toward diversifying your meals and promoting digestive comfort and well-being. Keep up the good work, and remember that patience and persistence are key as you continue on your journey toward recovery.

Week 3: Incorporating Balanced Nutrients

Congratulations on reaching Week 3 of your recovery journey! As your body continues to heal and adjust, it's time to focus on incorporating a well-rounded, nutrient-dense diet that provides the energy and nutrition needed for optimal recovery. This week is all about achieving balance by ensuring that your meals include a variety of macronutrients—carbohydrates, proteins, and fats—as well as essential vitamins and minerals.

Here's how to approach this important phase:

1. **Prioritize Lean Proteins:** Protein is vital for tissue repair and muscle maintenance, especially as your body recovers from surgery. Continue to include lean protein sources like chicken, turkey, fish, eggs, and tofu in your meals. You can also experiment with well-cooked beans and legumes, gradually introducing them in small amounts to assess your tolerance.

2. **Choose Complex Carbohydrates:** Carbohydrates are your body's main source of energy. This week, focus on including complex carbohydrates such as white rice, refined pasta, and well-cooked potatoes. These foods provide a steady release of energy and are easier to digest than whole grains.

3. **Incorporate Healthy Fats:** Healthy fats play a crucial role in hormone production, nutrient absorption, and overall cellular health. Include sources of healthy fats like olive oil, avocado, and soft margarine. If tolerated, small portions of nuts or seeds can be introduced, but be mindful of their fiber content.

4. **Include Cooked Vegetables and Fruits:** Expand your intake of cooked vegetables and fruits to ensure you're getting a range of vitamins and minerals. Try incorporating a wider variety of low-fiber vegetables, such as peeled zucchini, pumpkin, and parsnips, as well as fruits like peeled apples or ripe bananas. Avoid raw or fibrous varieties that may be harder to digest.

5. **Hydrate with Purpose:** Staying hydrated is crucial, especially when your ileostomy output can lead to increased fluid loss. Along with water, consider including electrolyte-rich fluids like broth, oral rehydration solutions, or diluted fruit juices to maintain electrolyte balance.

6. **Monitor and Adjust:** As you incorporate more balanced meals, pay close attention to your body's signals. Keep track of how different foods affect your digestion, energy levels, and overall well-being. If you experience discomfort, adjust your diet accordingly and consider consulting with a dietitian or healthcare provider.

This week is about finding the right mix of nutrients that works for your body, supporting not just your recovery but your overall health. By focusing on balanced meals that are rich in essential nutrients, you're laying the groundwork for sustained healing and long-term vitality. Remember, this is a journey, and finding what nourishes you best is a process of gradual exploration and mindful choices. Keep progressing, and embrace the diversity and balance in your diet as a pathway to wellness.

Week 4: Exploring Flavorful Options

Welcome to Week 4 of your ileostomy recovery plan! As you continue to heal and grow more comfortable with your dietary adjustments, it's time to bring some excitement and variety back into your meals by exploring flavorful options. This week focuses on reintroducing taste, spices, and textures into your diet while still being mindful of your body's unique needs.

Here's how to approach this flavorful phase:

1. **Introduce Mild Spices and Herbs:** Flavor doesn't have to mean heavy spices. Start with mild, non-irritating seasonings like basil, oregano, parsley, and dill. These herbs add fresh and vibrant flavors to your dishes without overwhelming your digestive system. Avoid hot spices like chili powder or cayenne, as they may cause irritation or discomfort.

2. **Experiment with New Cooking Techniques:** Diversify your meals by trying different cooking methods, such as grilling, baking, or steaming. These techniques can enhance the natural flavors

of your foods without the need for excessive seasoning or oils. Lightly sautéing vegetables or proteins can also introduce new textures and tastes while keeping your meals easily digestible.

3. **Incorporate Tolerable Flavors:** If your body is responding well, consider adding small amounts of flavorful ingredients like lemon juice, ginger, or a splash of balsamic vinegar. These can brighten up your meals without compromising your comfort. Start with small quantities to gauge your tolerance.

4. **Enhance Texture Gradually:** Along with flavor, texture plays a key role in meal satisfaction. Begin to reintroduce foods with slightly more texture, such as tender cooked meats, soft breads, or creamy casseroles. Avoid anything too crunchy or fibrous, as these could be difficult to digest.

5. **Explore Dairy Alternatives:** If dairy has been part of your diet, you can now try reintroducing small amounts of stronger-flavored cheeses like cheddar or feta, or enjoy flavored yogurts (watching for added sugars and fat). If you're lactose intolerant, consider trying lactose-free options or plant-based alternatives like almond or oat milk.

6. **Mindful Enjoyment:** As you explore new flavors and textures, continue to eat slowly and chew thoroughly. Pay attention to how your body reacts

to different foods, and make adjustments as needed. This week is about rediscovering the joy of eating while ensuring that your meals remain nourishing and supportive of your recovery.

Week 4 is a time to bring creativity and enjoyment back into your meals, making your dining experience more pleasurable while still keeping your health in check. By carefully reintroducing flavors and textures, you'll not only keep your taste buds engaged but also maintain the balance and nutrition necessary for ongoing healing. Embrace this week as an opportunity to rediscover your culinary preferences and to enjoy food as a source of both nourishment and delight.

Week 5: Enhancing Variety and Texture

You've reached Week 5 of your ileostomy recovery journey, and by now, your body is likely adjusting well to the changes you've made. This week is all about expanding your diet by introducing even more variety and texture. As you continue to heal, it's important to diversify your meals, both to prevent monotony and to ensure you're getting a wide range of nutrients.

Here's how to enhance variety and texture in your diet this week:

1. **Introduce Whole Grains Cautiously:** If you've been sticking to refined grains, now is the time to cautiously introduce more whole grains like brown rice, oatmeal, or quinoa in small portions. These grains add a nutty flavor and a firmer texture, providing more fiber while still being gentle on your digestive system. Be mindful of portion sizes to avoid overwhelming your digestive tract.

2. **Add More Raw Vegetables:** If your body has tolerated cooked vegetables well, you can begin to introduce small amounts of raw vegetables, starting with tender options like lettuce, cucumbers, or peeled tomatoes. These add a crisp texture and fresh flavor to your meals. Start with small portions and ensure they are well-chewed to ease digestion.

3. **Experiment with Nuts and Seeds:** For those who are ready, small quantities of finely chopped nuts or seeds can be introduced. They add a satisfying crunch and healthy fats to your meals. Be cautious with portions, and consider starting with nut butters if you're unsure about tolerating whole nuts.

4. **Incorporate More Protein Varieties:** Expand your protein options by trying different types of lean meats, fish, or plant-based proteins like tempeh or lentils (well-cooked). These provide

diverse flavors and textures, helping you to meet your protein needs while keeping your meals interesting.

5. **Try Different Dairy Products:** If you've been eating soft dairy products like yogurt and cottage cheese, you might now try harder cheeses or a wider variety of dairy alternatives, like flavored nut milks or kefir. These add new textures and tastes to your diet, allowing for greater diversity.

6. **Increase Portion Sizes Gradually:** As you introduce more variety, you may also start to increase your portion sizes slightly if your body is responding well. This helps to ensure that you're getting enough calories and nutrients to support your continued healing and energy needs.

Throughout Week 5, continue to be mindful of your body's signals as you incorporate new foods. Keeping a food journal can help you track how different textures and varieties affect your digestion and overall well-being. Remember to chew thoroughly, eat slowly, and stay hydrated to support your digestive process.

By enhancing variety and texture in your diet, you're taking an important step toward normalizing your eating habits and enjoying a more diverse, satisfying range of foods. This week is about embracing the richness and diversity of your meals, which not only nourishes your body but also keeps your culinary experience engaging and enjoyable. Keep exploring and savoring each new addition to your plate!

Week 6: Sustainable Diet for Long-Term Healing

Congratulations on reaching Week 6 of your ileostomy recovery journey! This final week of the recovery plan is focused on transitioning from a recovery-focused diet to a sustainable, long-term eating plan that will support your health and well-being for the years to come. The goal this week is to establish a diet that's not only nourishing but also enjoyable and sustainable, allowing you to live a full and vibrant life post-surgery.

Here's how to approach building a sustainable diet for long-term healing:

1. **Embrace a Balanced Diet:** By now, you've explored a variety of foods and found what works best for your body. Continue to focus on a balanced diet that includes a variety of fruits, vegetables, lean proteins, whole grains, and healthy fats. Balance is key to ensuring you receive all the essential nutrients your body needs to thrive.

2. **Personalize Your Food Choices:** Over the past five weeks, you've learned a lot about your body's unique responses to different foods. Use this knowledge to personalize your diet, including the foods you enjoy and that make you feel good. Whether it's incorporating more plant-based meals, enjoying lean meats, or experimenting with different grains, your diet should reflect your preferences and nutritional needs.

3. **Manage Portions and Frequency:** With a focus on sustainability, it's important to manage portion sizes and meal frequency in a way that works for your lifestyle. Eating smaller, more frequent meals can help with digestion and energy levels, while ensuring you're meeting your nutritional needs without overwhelming your digestive system.

4. **Stay Hydrated:** Maintaining proper hydration remains crucial, especially as you settle into your long-term diet. Continue to drink plenty of water, and consider including hydrating foods like soups, smoothies, and water-rich fruits and vegetables in your meals.

5. **Incorporate Regular Physical Activity:** As part of a sustainable lifestyle, consider incorporating regular physical activity that complements your diet. Gentle exercises like walking, swimming, or

yoga can aid digestion, improve mood, and support overall health.

6. **Monitor and Adjust as Needed:** Life with an ileostomy is an ongoing journey, and your dietary needs may evolve over time. Regularly assess how you're feeling, and be prepared to adjust your diet as needed to accommodate changes in your health, activity level, or any new dietary preferences that emerge.

7. **Enjoy the Journey:** The most important aspect of a sustainable diet is that it's enjoyable and fulfilling. Continue to experiment with new recipes, explore different cuisines, and share meals with loved ones. Eating should be a source of pleasure and nourishment, not just a necessity.

By the end of Week 6, you'll have developed a diet that's tailored to your body's needs and preferences, setting you up for long-term success and well-being. This sustainable approach will help you maintain your health, manage your ileostomy with confidence, and enjoy a vibrant, fulfilling life. Remember, this is just the beginning—continue to listen to your body, make informed choices, and embrace the journey ahead with positivity and resilience.

Chapter 3: Essential Tips for Cooking and Meal Preparation

In this chapter, we'll dive into practical tips and strategies to make your cooking and meal preparation not only manageable but enjoyable. Adapting to life with an ileostomy doesn't mean sacrificing delicious meals or spending endless hours in the kitchen. With the right tools, planning, and techniques, you can create satisfying, nutritious meals that support your health and recovery. This chapter will guide you through essential kitchen tools, smart meal planning, safe cooking techniques, and pantry essentials, all tailored to the unique needs of ileostomy patients.

Kitchen Essentials for Ileostomy Patients

Setting up a kitchen that caters to your specific dietary needs is the first step in making meal preparation enjoyable and stress-free. Having the right tools and gadgets on hand can simplify the process of creating meals that are both gentle on your digestive system and satisfying to eat. Below are some essential kitchen items that every ileostomy patient should consider having:

1. Blender or Food Processor

A high-quality blender or food processor is invaluable for preparing smoothies, purees, and soups. These appliances allow you to break down foods into easily digestible forms, which is especially important in the early stages of your recovery when soft, smooth textures are recommended.

2. Steamer Basket or Steamer Pot

Steaming is one of the best cooking methods for retaining the nutrients in your food while ensuring that vegetables and proteins are soft and easy to digest. A steamer basket or a dedicated steamer pot makes it simple to cook vegetables, fish, and even poultry in a way that's gentle on your digestive system.

3. Slow Cooker or Instant Pot

These versatile appliances can be lifesavers for anyone with a busy schedule. Slow cookers and Instant Pots allow you to prepare nutrient-rich meals with minimal effort. You can cook stews, soups, and casseroles that are tender and flavorful, all while freeing up your time for other activities.

4. Fine Mesh Strainer or Sieve

A fine mesh strainer is essential for preparing foods that need to be drained of excess liquid or for making purees and soups that require a smooth consistency. It's also useful for rinsing small grains, like quinoa, to ensure they're soft and easy to digest.

5. Soft Spatulas and Utensils

Using soft, silicone spatulas and utensils can help you handle delicate foods without breaking them apart. These tools are particularly useful when preparing dishes like scrambled eggs or delicate fish that need to be cooked gently to retain their texture.

6. Sharp Knives and a Good Cutting Board

A set of sharp knives and a sturdy cutting board are essential for preparing your ingredients efficiently. Sharp knives make it easier to chop fruits, vegetables, and proteins into the small, manageable pieces that are ideal for easy digestion.

7. Storage Containers

Having a variety of storage containers on hand allows you to store prepped ingredients and leftovers safely. Choose containers that are airtight and easy to label, so you can quickly identify the contents and their preparation date. This makes meal planning and portion control much simpler.

8. Mashing Tools

Potato mashers or food mills can help you prepare mashed vegetables, fruits, and even proteins. These tools allow you to create smooth, lump-free dishes that are gentle on your digestive system, ideal for the early recovery stages.

9. Immersion Blender

An immersion blender is a handy tool for blending soups and sauces directly in the pot, saving you time and reducing the number of dishes to clean. It's perfect for creating smooth, creamy textures without transferring hot liquids to a blender.

10. Cooking Thermometer

Ensuring your food is cooked to the proper temperature is crucial for both safety and digestion. A cooking thermometer helps you verify that meats and other foods are cooked thoroughly, reducing the risk of digestive discomfort or infection.

By equipping your kitchen with these essential tools, you'll be better prepared to create meals that meet your dietary needs while also enjoying the process of cooking.

Smart Meal Planning Strategies

Meal planning is a powerful tool for anyone, but it's especially valuable for ileostomy patients who need to manage their diet carefully to ensure smooth digestion and overall well-being. By planning your meals in advance, you can make sure you're eating a balanced diet, reduce stress around meal times, and avoid last-minute decisions that might lead to discomfort. Here's how to implement smart meal planning strategies tailored to your needs:

1. Start with a Weekly Meal Plan

Begin by creating a weekly meal plan that outlines breakfast, lunch, dinner, and snacks for each day. Consider your energy levels, your schedule, and any specific dietary requirements you have. Planning for the week ahead helps you stay organized and ensures that you have all the necessary ingredients on hand.

- **Balance Your Meals:** Make sure each meal includes a balance of protein, carbohydrates, and healthy fats. This balance will help sustain your energy levels and support your recovery.
- **Include Variety:** To prevent boredom and ensure you're getting a wide range of nutrients, plan for different types of meals throughout the week. Rotate your protein sources (e.g., chicken, fish, tofu), vary your vegetables, and try different grains or starches.

2. Prep Ingredients in Advance

Once your meal plan is set, dedicate some time to prepping ingredients in advance. This can include washing and chopping vegetables, cooking grains, or marinating proteins. Prepping ahead of time saves you from doing everything at once and makes it easier to throw together a healthy meal when you're short on time or energy.

- **Batch Cooking:** Cook larger portions of grains, proteins, or soups that can be stored in the fridge or freezer and used throughout the week. This method is efficient and ensures you always have something healthy to eat.
- **Portion Control:** Use your prep time to portion out meals and snacks into individual containers. This not only helps with managing your food intake but also makes it easier to grab a meal or snack when you're on the go.

3. Plan for Flexibility

While having a plan is important, it's also essential to remain flexible. Some days you may not feel like eating what you've planned, or you might have leftovers that need to be used up. Build flexibility into your meal plan by having a few go-to meals or ingredients that can be quickly prepared if plans change.

- **Quick and Easy Meals:** Keep a few simple, quick-to-make meals in your rotation for days when you're too tired or busy to cook. These could be something as simple as scrambled eggs with toast or a smoothie with a protein source.
- **Leftover Days:** Plan for one or two days a week where you use up leftovers. This reduces food waste and saves you from cooking another meal.

4. Shop with a Purpose

Based on your meal plan, create a detailed shopping list that includes everything you need for the week. Shopping with a list helps you stay focused, ensures you don't forget any key ingredients, and helps avoid impulse buys that might not fit into your dietary plan.

- **Stick to the Perimeter:** The perimeter of the grocery store typically houses fresh produce, dairy, and meats—key components of a healthy diet. Focus your shopping here and avoid the aisles with processed foods as much as possible.

- **Check Labels:** When purchasing packaged foods, take the time to read labels to ensure they meet your dietary requirements, especially concerning fiber content, additives, and any potential irritants.

5. Incorporate Snacks Wisely

Snacks can be an important part of your diet, especially if you need to eat smaller meals more frequently. Plan for healthy, easy-to-digest snacks that you can enjoy between meals to keep your energy levels stable.

- **Easy Snacks:** Consider snacks like yogurt, a small portion of soft fruit, or nut butter on white bread. These snacks are not only convenient but also gentle on your digestive system.

- **Pre-Portioned Snacks:** Prepare snacks in advance by portioning them into small containers or bags.

This helps with portion control and ensures you have a ready-to-eat option whenever you need it.

6. Listen to Your Body

Finally, it's important to listen to your body and adjust your meal plan as needed. Some foods that work well for others might not suit you, and that's okay. Pay attention to how different meals make you feel, and don't be afraid to tweak your plan if something isn't working.

- **Keep a Food Journal:** Tracking what you eat and how you feel afterward can help you identify patterns and make informed decisions about your diet. This can be particularly helpful if you're trying to figure out which foods are easiest on your system.

- **Adjust for Your Needs:** If you find that certain meals are too heavy or don't sit well, adjust your plan to include more of the foods that work best for you.

Safe Cooking Techniques for Easy Digestion

Cooking techniques play a crucial role in how well your body can digest and absorb the nutrients from your food, especially after an ileostomy. Certain methods can make food easier to digest, reduce the risk of blockages, and ensure that you're getting the most out of your meals. In this section, we'll explore safe and effective cooking techniques that are particularly beneficial for ileostomy patients.

1. Steaming

Steaming is one of the best cooking methods for preserving nutrients while also making food tender and easy to digest. It's ideal for vegetables, fish, and even some fruits.

- **How to Steam:** Use a steamer basket placed over a pot of boiling water, or invest in an electric steamer. Ensure that the food is cooked until it's soft and tender, which makes it easier to break down in your digestive system.

- **Benefits:** Steaming helps retain the vitamins and minerals in your food, avoids the need for added fats, and produces a soft texture that's gentle on your digestive tract.

2. Boiling and Simmering

Boiling and simmering are simple, effective methods for cooking foods like vegetables, grains, and proteins. These techniques soften the food, making it easier to chew and digest.

- **How to Boil/Simmer:** Bring water or broth to a boil, then reduce the heat to a simmer and cook until the food is tender. For added flavor, use a low-sodium broth instead of plain water.

- **Benefits:** Boiling and simmering allow you to prepare foods that are easy to digest and absorb. These methods also make it easy to prepare large batches of soups or stews that can be stored and reheated.

3. Slow Cooking

A slow cooker is an excellent tool for preparing tender, flavorful meals without much effort. Slow cooking allows foods to cook gently over several hours, breaking down tough fibers and making them easier to digest.

- **How to Slow Cook:** Place your ingredients in a slow cooker with enough liquid to cover them. Cook on low for 6-8 hours or on high for 3-4 hours, depending on the recipe. The result is tender, well-cooked food that's gentle on your digestive system.

- **Benefits:** Slow cooking is convenient and produces meals that are soft and full of flavor. It's particularly good for preparing meats, beans, and root vegetables that might otherwise be too tough or fibrous.

4. Blanching

Blanching is a technique that involves briefly boiling food, then plunging it into ice water to stop the cooking process. This method is often used to prepare vegetables, making them tender yet crisp and preserving their bright color.

- **How to Blanch:** Bring a pot of water to a boil, add the vegetables, and cook for 1-3 minutes, depending on their size. Immediately transfer the vegetables to a bowl of ice water to cool them quickly.
- **Benefits:** Blanching softens vegetables slightly while retaining their nutrients and flavor. It's a great way to prepare vegetables that you want to use in salads, stir-fries, or as a side dish.

5. Baking and Roasting

Baking and roasting are versatile cooking methods that can be used for a wide variety of foods, including vegetables, proteins, and grains. These methods allow you to cook food evenly while enhancing natural flavors.

- **How to Bake/Roast:** Preheat your oven and place the food on a baking sheet or in a roasting pan. Cook until the food is golden and tender. For added moisture, cover the dish with foil or add a bit of broth or water to the pan.
- **Benefits:** Baking and roasting concentrate the flavors of your food without the need for excess fat

or oil. When done properly, these methods produce tender, easy-to-digest meals.

6. Poaching

Poaching is a gentle cooking technique that involves simmering food in liquid just below boiling. It's ideal for delicate proteins like fish, chicken, or eggs.

- **How to Poach:** Fill a pan with water, broth, or another flavorful liquid, and bring it to a gentle simmer. Add the food and cook until it's done, usually just a few minutes for fish or eggs.
- **Benefits:** Poaching is a low-fat cooking method that keeps food moist and tender. It's particularly good for creating soft, easily digestible meals that are still full of flavor.

7. Pureeing

Pureeing involves blending or processing food into a smooth, thick consistency. This method is particularly useful for making soups, smoothies, and sauces that are easy to swallow and digest.

- **How to Puree:** Use a blender, food processor, or immersion blender to puree cooked foods until smooth. You can add liquid (such as broth, milk, or water) to achieve the desired consistency.
- **Benefits:** Pureeing is perfect for creating meals that are gentle on your digestive system, especially

in the early stages of recovery. It allows you to enjoy a variety of foods in a form that's easy to digest.

8. Avoiding Frying

While frying can add flavor and texture to foods, it's generally not recommended for ileostomy patients, as it can make food difficult to digest and increase the risk of irritation.

- **Alternative Methods:** Instead of frying, opt for baking, steaming, or poaching, which produce similar results without the added fat and potential digestive discomfort.
- **Benefits:** By avoiding frying, you reduce the risk of indigestion, bloating, and other issues that can arise from consuming too much fat or oil.

By focusing on these safe cooking techniques, you can prepare meals that are not only delicious but also easy on your digestive system.

Stocking Your Pantry with Ileostomy-Friendly Ingredients

Having a well-stocked pantry is key to making meal preparation easier and ensuring that you always have ileostomy-friendly options on hand. By choosing ingredients that are gentle on your digestive system, you can create a variety of delicious meals that support your recovery and long-term health. Below is a guide to essential pantry items that every ileostomy patient should consider keeping in stock.

1. Low-Fiber Grains

Grains are a staple in many diets, and selecting the right types is crucial for ease of digestion. Low-fiber options are preferable as they reduce the risk of blockages and irritation.

- **White Rice:** A gentle, easily digestible option that serves as a versatile base for many meals.

- **Pasta:** Choose refined pasta made from white flour, which is lower in fiber and easier on the digestive system.

- **White Bread:** Soft, white bread is easier to digest than whole grain varieties and can be used in sandwiches, toast, or as a side with meals.

- **Oatmeal (Smooth or Instant):** Choose smooth or instant oatmeal, which is lower in fiber compared to steel-cut oats, and easy to prepare.
- **Polenta:** This ground cornmeal is a versatile option that can be served as a soft porridge or allowed to set and sliced.

2. Lean Proteins

Protein is essential for healing and maintaining muscle mass, especially after surgery. Lean proteins are easier to digest and can be prepared in a variety of ways.

- **Chicken Breast:** Skinless chicken breast is a lean source of protein that's versatile and easy to digest.
- **Turkey:** Ground turkey or turkey breast offers a lean alternative to beef and can be used in many recipes.
- **Fish:** White fish like cod, haddock, or tilapia are low in fat and easy on the digestive system. Canned tuna or salmon packed in water are convenient options as well.
- **Eggs:** Eggs are a soft, easily digestible source of protein that can be prepared in numerous ways, from scrambled to poached.
- **Tofu:** A plant-based protein that's soft and easy to digest, tofu is an excellent option for vegetarian meals.

3. Fruits and Vegetables

While fruits and vegetables are essential for a balanced diet, it's important to choose varieties that are low in fiber and easy to digest.

- **Canned or Cooked Vegetables:** Opt for peeled, cooked, or canned vegetables such as carrots, green beans, and pumpkin. Avoid raw or fibrous vegetables like broccoli and cabbage.
- **Peeled Potatoes:** Potatoes (white or sweet) without skins are a starchy, gentle option that can be baked, mashed, or boiled.
- **Bananas:** Soft, ripe bananas are an excellent fruit choice that is low in fiber and easy on the digestive system.
- **Applesauce:** Unsweetened applesauce provides a gentle source of fruit that's easy to digest. Make sure it's smooth and free from chunks.
- **Avocado:** Although slightly higher in fat, avocado is smooth, creamy, and generally well-tolerated in small amounts.

4. Dairy and Dairy Alternatives

Dairy can be a good source of calcium and protein, but it's important to choose options that are easy to digest.

- **Lactose-Free Milk:** Some ileostomy patients find that lactose-free milk is easier to digest than regular milk.

- **Yogurt (Without Fruit Pieces):** Choose plain or vanilla yogurt that's smooth and free of fruit chunks or seeds. Greek yogurt is also a good option for higher protein content.

- **Cheese:** Soft cheeses like mozzarella or cottage cheese are generally well-tolerated and can be used in various dishes.

- **Almond Milk or Other Non-Dairy Milks:** If you prefer to avoid dairy, almond milk or other non-dairy alternatives can be used in cooking and baking.

5. Healthy Fats

Healthy fats are essential for energy and overall health, but they should be consumed in moderation and in easily digestible forms.

- **Olive Oil:** A heart-healthy fat that can be used for cooking or drizzling over dishes.

- **Coconut Oil:** Another easily digestible oil that can be used in cooking or baking.

- **Smooth Nut Butters:** Choose smooth peanut butter or almond butter, which can be spread on toast or added to smoothies.

6. Broths and Soups

Broths and soups are comforting, hydrating, and easy to digest, making them ideal for ileostomy patients.

- **Low-Sodium Broth:** Chicken, beef, or vegetable broth can be used as a base for soups or as a way to cook grains and proteins.

- **Creamy Soups:** Opt for smooth, creamy soups without chunks of vegetables or meat. You can make your own or choose store-bought versions that are low in fiber.

7. Hydration Essentials

Staying hydrated is crucial for ileostomy patients, so it's important to have hydration options readily available.

- **Electrolyte Drinks:** Keep electrolyte drinks on hand to help maintain hydration, especially if you've had high output from your ileostomy.

- **Herbal Teas:** Caffeine-free herbal teas can be soothing and hydrating. Choose teas that are gentle on the stomach, like chamomile or peppermint.

- **Coconut Water:** A natural source of electrolytes, coconut water can be a refreshing and hydrating option.

8. Digestive Aids

Certain ingredients can help support digestion and prevent discomfort.

- **Ginger:** Fresh or powdered ginger can be used to make tea or add flavor to dishes, helping to soothe the digestive tract.
- **Probiotic Supplements:** Consider keeping probiotic supplements that support gut health and aid digestion.

9. Flavor Enhancers

Flavor doesn't have to be sacrificed for easy digestion. Stock your pantry with gentle, flavor-enhancing ingredients.

- **Herbs and Spices:** Mild herbs like basil, parsley, and oregano can add flavor without irritating the digestive system. Avoid spicy or heavily seasoned options.
- **Lemon Juice:** A splash of lemon juice can brighten up flavors without being too harsh on the stomach.
- **Low-Sodium Soy Sauce:** Use soy sauce in moderation to add umami flavor to dishes without adding too much salt.

By stocking your pantry with these ileostomy-friendly ingredients, you'll be well-prepared to create meals that are both nourishing and easy on your digestive system.

These essentials will not only help you stick to a safe and healthy diet but also make meal preparation simpler and more enjoyable, allowing you to focus on your recovery and long-term well-being.

Chapter 4: Breakfast Recipes for a Nourishing Start

10 Energizing Smoothies and Shakes

Smoothies and shakes are excellent breakfast options for ileostomy patients, providing essential nutrients in a form that's easy to digest. They're versatile, quick to prepare, and can be tailored to meet your specific dietary needs. Here's a selection of 10 energizing smoothies and shakes that will help you start your day on the right foot.

1. Banana-Oat Smoothie

- **Ingredients:** 1 ripe banana, ½ cup smooth oats (cooked), 1 cup lactose-free milk or almond milk, 1 tablespoon smooth peanut butter, 1 teaspoon honey.

- **Preparation:** Blend all ingredients until smooth. Serve chilled.

- **Benefits:** This smoothie provides a balance of carbohydrates, protein, and healthy fats, making it a filling and energizing breakfast option.

2. Berry-Almond Protein Shake

- **Ingredients:** 1 cup mixed berries (strawberries, blueberries), 1 scoop vanilla protein powder, 1 cup almond milk, 1 tablespoon almond butter, ½ teaspoon vanilla extract.

- **Preparation:** Blend until smooth and enjoy immediately.
- **Benefits:** Packed with antioxidants from the berries and protein from the powder and almond butter, this shake supports muscle recovery and overall health.

3. Tropical Mango Smoothie

- **Ingredients:** 1 cup frozen mango chunks, ½ cup plain yogurt, 1 cup coconut water, 1 tablespoon chia seeds (soaked), 1 teaspoon lime juice.
- **Preparation:** Blend all ingredients until smooth. Serve with a slice of lime.
- **Benefits:** This tropical smoothie is hydrating and rich in vitamins, making it a refreshing and nutrient-dense start to your day.

4. Creamy Avocado and Spinach Shake

- **Ingredients:** ½ ripe avocado, 1 handful of spinach (optional), 1 banana, 1 cup lactose-free milk, 1 tablespoon honey.
- **Preparation:** Blend until creamy and smooth. Serve immediately.

- **Benefits:** Avocado adds creaminess and healthy fats, while spinach provides a mild dose of greens that's easy on your digestive system.

5. Peach and Greek Yogurt Smoothie

- **Ingredients:** 1 cup ripe peaches (peeled and sliced), ½ cup Greek yogurt, 1 tablespoon honey, 1 cup almond milk, 1 teaspoon vanilla extract.
- **Preparation:** Blend until smooth. Optionally, add ice for a chilled version.
- **Benefits:** This smoothie offers a delicious blend of protein and vitamins, perfect for a light yet satisfying breakfast.

6. Apple Cinnamon Breakfast Shake

- **Ingredients:** 1 apple (peeled and sliced), ½ cup smooth oats (cooked), 1 cup lactose-free milk, 1 teaspoon cinnamon, 1 tablespoon almond butter.
- **Preparation:** Blend all ingredients until smooth. Serve with a sprinkle of cinnamon.
- **Benefits:** The combination of apple and cinnamon provides a comforting flavor while oats and almond butter offer sustained energy.

7. Strawberry Banana Power Smoothie

- **Ingredients:** 1 banana, 1 cup strawberries, 1 scoop vanilla protein powder, 1 cup almond milk, 1 teaspoon honey.

- **Preparation:** Blend until smooth and creamy. Serve immediately.

- **Benefits:** This classic smoothie is a powerhouse of vitamins and protein, perfect for a post-workout breakfast or a morning energy boost.

8. Chocolate Peanut Butter Shake

- **Ingredients:** 1 scoop chocolate protein powder, 1 tablespoon smooth peanut butter, 1 banana, 1 cup lactose-free milk, 1 teaspoon honey.

- **Preparation:** Blend until smooth. Enjoy as a rich, indulgent treat.

- **Benefits:** This shake offers a delicious blend of chocolate and peanut butter flavors while providing protein and healthy fats.

9. Melon and Mint Smoothie

- **Ingredients:** 1 cup cantaloupe or honeydew melon (cubed), 1 cup coconut water, 1 tablespoon fresh mint leaves, 1 teaspoon honey.

- **Preparation:** Blend until smooth. Serve with a mint garnish.

- **Benefits:** Refreshing and hydrating, this smoothie is light on the stomach and perfect for hot days.

10. Vanilla Chai Breakfast Shake

- **Ingredients:** 1 scoop vanilla protein powder, 1 cup lactose-free milk, 1 teaspoon chai spice mix, 1 tablespoon honey, ½ banana (optional).
- **Preparation:** Blend all ingredients until smooth. Serve chilled.
- **Benefits:** This shake provides the warm, spiced flavors of chai combined with the nutrition of a balanced breakfast shake.

10 Soft and Easily Digestible Breakfast Bowls

1. Creamy Rice Porridge

- **Ingredients:**
    - 1 cup cooked white rice
    - 1 cup lactose-free milk
    - 1 tablespoon honey
    - A pinch of cinnamon
- **Instructions:**

1. In a small pot, combine the cooked rice and lactose-free milk.

2. Simmer over low heat, stirring occasionally, until the mixture becomes creamy.

3. Stir in the honey and cinnamon.

4. Serve warm.

- **Benefits:**
    - This porridge is soothing and easy on the digestive system, providing sustained energy with minimal strain.

2. Mashed Banana and Oat Bowl

- **Ingredients:**

- ½ cup smooth oats (cooked)
- 1 ripe banana, mashed
- 1 tablespoon almond butter
- A drizzle of honey

- **Instructions:**

1. In a bowl, combine the cooked oats and mashed banana.
2. Stir in the almond butter and drizzle with honey.
3. Mix until well combined and serve warm.

- **Benefits:**
  - This bowl offers a balance of carbohydrates and healthy fats, making it a satisfying and gentle breakfast.

3. Soft Polenta with Yogurt and Honey

- **Ingredients:**
  - ½ cup polenta (cooked)
  - ¼ cup Greek yogurt
  - 1 tablespoon honey
  - A pinch of cinnamon
- **Instructions:**

1. Cook the polenta according to package instructions until smooth.

2. Top with Greek yogurt, honey, and a pinch of cinnamon.

3. Serve warm.

- **Benefits:**
    - Rich in protein, this bowl is creamy and comforting, perfect for easy digestion.

4. Pumpkin Spice Quinoa Bowl

- **Ingredients:**
    - ½ cup cooked quinoa
    - ¼ cup pumpkin puree
    - 1 tablespoon honey
    - A pinch of pumpkin pie spice
- **Instructions:**

1. Combine cooked quinoa and pumpkin puree in a bowl.

2. Stir in honey and pumpkin pie spice.

3. Mix well and serve warm.

- **Benefits:**

- Quinoa provides complete protein, while pumpkin adds a gentle, digestible fiber and sweetness.

5. Soft Scrambled Eggs with Avocado

- **Ingredients:**
  - 2 eggs
  - ½ avocado, sliced
  - 1 slice soft white bread, toasted
  - A pinch of salt
- **Instructions:**

1. Crack the eggs into a bowl and whisk until well blended.
2. In a non-stick pan, cook the eggs over low heat, stirring gently until soft and creamy.
3. Serve the eggs on the toasted bread, topped with avocado slices and a pinch of salt.

- **Benefits:**
  - This bowl is rich in protein and healthy fats, making it easy to digest and energy-sustaining.

6. Apple Cinnamon Oat Bowl

- **Ingredients:**

- ½ cup smooth oats (cooked)
- ½ apple, peeled and diced
- 1 teaspoon cinnamon
- 1 tablespoon honey

- **Instructions:**

1. Prepare the oats according to package instructions.
2. Stir in the diced apple, cinnamon, and honey.
3. Mix well and serve warm.

- **Benefits:**
  - This comforting bowl is rich in gentle fiber and flavor, perfect for a nourishing start to the day.

7. Peach and Cottage Cheese Bowl

- **Ingredients:**
  - 1 cup cottage cheese
  - ½ cup canned peaches, sliced
  - 1 tablespoon honey

- **Instructions:**

1. In a bowl, combine the cottage cheese and peach slices.
2. Drizzle with honey.

3. Mix gently and serve chilled.
- **Benefits:**
  - This bowl offers a soft texture and a balance of protein and fruit, making it easy on the digestive system.

8. Creamy Grits with Soft Boiled Egg

- **Ingredients:**
  - ½ cup grits (cooked)
  - 1 soft-boiled egg
  - A pinch of salt and pepper
- **Instructions:**

1. Cook the grits according to package instructions until creamy.
2. Peel the soft-boiled egg and place it on top of the grits.
3. Season with salt and pepper.
4. Serve warm.

- **Benefits:**
  - Grits are easy to digest, and the addition of a soft-boiled egg provides gentle protein.

9. Smoothie Bowl

- **Ingredients:**
    - 1 banana
    - ½ cup Greek yogurt
    - ½ cup lactose-free milk
    - 1 tablespoon honey
- **Instructions:**

1. Blend the banana, Greek yogurt, lactose-free milk, and honey until smooth.

2. Pour into a bowl and enjoy immediately.

- **Benefits:**
    - This smoothie bowl is rich in protein and easy to digest, providing a refreshing and nutritious breakfast.

10. Blueberry Vanilla Oatmeal

- **Ingredients:**
    - ½ cup smooth oats (cooked)
    - ¼ cup blueberries (fresh or cooked)
    - 1 teaspoon vanilla extract
    - 1 tablespoon honey
- **Instructions:**

1. Cook the oats according to package instructions.

2. Stir in the blueberries, vanilla extract, and honey.
3. Serve warm.
- **Benefits:**
    - Blueberries add antioxidants, while vanilla and honey provide a gentle sweetness, making this bowl a delicious and nutritious choice.

10 Creative Egg Dishes and Alternatives

Eggs are a versatile and easy-to-digest source of protein, making them an ideal choice for those recovering from ileostomy surgery. Here are 10 creative ways to enjoy eggs and alternatives that are gentle on your digestive system.

1. Herbed Egg Scramble

- **Ingredients:**
    - 2 eggs
    - 1 tablespoon lactose-free milk
    - 1 teaspoon chopped fresh herbs (like parsley or chives)
    - A pinch of salt and pepper

- **Instructions:**

1. Crack the eggs into a bowl, add the milk, and whisk until well combined.

2. Pour the mixture into a non-stick pan over low heat, stirring gently until the eggs are soft and scrambled.

3. Sprinkle with fresh herbs, salt, and pepper before serving.

- **Benefits:**
  - This dish is light, protein-rich, and packed with the fresh flavor of herbs, making it an excellent and easy-to-digest option.

2. Baked Egg Cups

- **Ingredients:**
  - 4 eggs
  - ½ cup lactose-free cheese, shredded
  - ¼ cup finely diced bell peppers
  - ¼ cup cooked spinach (optional)
  - A pinch of salt and pepper
- **Instructions:**

1. Preheat the oven to 350°F (175°C).

2. Grease a muffin tin and evenly distribute the bell peppers and spinach into four cups.

3. Crack an egg into each cup, sprinkle with cheese, and season with salt and pepper.

4. Bake for 15-20 minutes, or until the eggs are set.

5. Serve warm.

- **Benefits:**
  - These portable egg cups are packed with protein and can be made in advance, offering a convenient and nourishing breakfast option.

3. Soft Boiled Eggs with Toast Soldiers

- **Ingredients:**
  - 2 eggs
  - 2 slices soft white bread
  - A pinch of salt and pepper
- **Instructions:**

1. Boil water in a small pot and carefully add the eggs.

2. Cook for 5-6 minutes, then remove the eggs and cool slightly.

3. While the eggs cook, toast the bread and cut it into strips (soldiers).

4. Serve the soft-boiled eggs with the toast soldiers for dipping.

- **Benefits:**
  - This classic dish is comforting and easy to digest, providing a simple yet satisfying breakfast.

4. Spinach and Feta Omelette

- **Ingredients:**
  - 2 eggs
  - ¼ cup cooked spinach, finely chopped
  - 2 tablespoons lactose-free feta cheese, crumbled
  - 1 teaspoon olive oil
  - A pinch of salt and pepper
- **Instructions:**

1. In a bowl, whisk the eggs until frothy.

2. Heat olive oil in a non-stick pan over medium heat, then pour in the eggs.

3. As the eggs begin to set, sprinkle the spinach and feta over one side.

4. Fold the omelette in half and cook until the eggs are fully set.

5. Serve warm with a pinch of salt and pepper.

- **Benefits:**
    - This omelette is packed with protein and leafy greens, offering a nutrient-dense start to your day.

5. Egg White and Cheese Roll-Up

- **Ingredients:**
    - 3 egg whites
    - ¼ cup lactose-free cheese, shredded
    - 1 teaspoon olive oil
    - A pinch of salt and pepper
- **Instructions:**

1. Whisk the egg whites with a pinch of salt and pepper.

2. Heat olive oil in a non-stick pan over medium heat.

3. Pour in the egg whites, swirling to coat the pan evenly.

4. Cook until the egg whites are set, then sprinkle with cheese.

5. Roll up the egg white like a burrito and serve warm.

- **Benefits:**

- This light and protein-rich dish is gentle on the stomach and can be prepared quickly, making it perfect for busy mornings.

6. Zucchini and Egg Frittata

- **Ingredients:**
    - 2 eggs
    - ½ cup zucchini, thinly sliced
    - 1 tablespoon olive oil
    - 2 tablespoons lactose-free cheese, shredded
    - A pinch of salt and pepper
- **Instructions:**

1. Preheat the oven to 350°F (175°C).
2. In a small oven-safe pan, heat the olive oil over medium heat.
3. Add the zucchini slices and cook until tender.
4. In a bowl, whisk the eggs with salt and pepper, then pour over the zucchini.
5. Sprinkle with cheese and transfer the pan to the oven.
6. Bake for 10-12 minutes, or until the eggs are fully set.
7. Serve warm.

- **Benefits:**
    - This frittata is a filling and nutritious dish that combines protein with vegetables in a way that's easy on digestion.

7. Egg and Avocado Toast

- **Ingredients:**
    - 1 egg
    - ½ avocado, mashed
    - 1 slice soft white bread, toasted
    - A pinch of salt and pepper
- **Instructions:**

1. Cook the egg to your preferred style (fried, poached, or scrambled).

2. Spread the mashed avocado on the toasted bread.

3. Top with the egg and season with salt and pepper.

4. Serve immediately.

- **Benefits:**
    - This dish combines protein, healthy fats, and fiber, offering a balanced and nourishing breakfast option.

8. Egg Salad with Greek Yogurt

- **Ingredients:**
    - 2 hard-boiled eggs, chopped
    - 2 tablespoons Greek yogurt
    - 1 teaspoon Dijon mustard
    - 1 tablespoon fresh chives, chopped
    - A pinch of salt and pepper
- **Instructions:**

1. In a bowl, combine the chopped eggs, Greek yogurt, and Dijon mustard.

2. Mix in the fresh chives and season with salt and pepper.

3. Serve on its own or spread on soft bread.

- **Benefits:**
    - This egg salad is creamy and packed with protein, but lighter than traditional versions thanks to the Greek yogurt.

9. Tofu Scramble

- **Ingredients:**
    - ½ block firm tofu, crumbled
    - 1 tablespoon olive oil
    - 1 teaspoon turmeric

- ¼ teaspoon cumin
- A pinch of salt and pepper

- **Instructions:**

1. Heat olive oil in a non-stick pan over medium heat.
2. Add the crumbled tofu, turmeric, and cumin, and cook until heated through, stirring occasionally.
3. Season with salt and pepper and serve warm.

- **Benefits:**
  - This egg alternative is high in protein and offers a flavorful, plant-based option for those who prefer or need a substitute for eggs.

10. Egg Custard

- **Ingredients:**
  - 2 eggs
  - 1 cup lactose-free milk
  - 2 tablespoons honey
  - 1 teaspoon vanilla extract

- **Instructions:**

1. Preheat the oven to 325°F (160°C).

2. In a bowl, whisk together the eggs, lactose-free milk, honey, and vanilla extract.

3. Pour the mixture into ramekins or a small baking dish.

4. Place the ramekins in a baking pan filled with about an inch of water.

5. Bake for 30-35 minutes, or until the custard is set.

6. Let cool slightly before serving.

- **Benefits:**
    - This smooth and creamy custard is gentle on the digestive system, making it a perfect breakfast or dessert option.

10 Quick Grab-and-Go Options

For busy mornings when you need something quick yet nourishing, these grab-and-go breakfast options are perfect. They are designed to be easy on the stomach while providing essential nutrients to start your day right.

1. Banana and Almond Butter Wrap

- **Ingredients:**
    - 1 soft whole-wheat tortilla
    - 1 ripe banana
    - 2 tablespoons almond butter
- **Instructions:**

1. Spread almond butter evenly on the tortilla.
2. Place the banana in the center and wrap the tortilla around it.
3. Cut in half and enjoy on the go.

- **Benefits:**
    - This wrap is quick to prepare and provides a balanced combination of carbohydrates, protein, and healthy fats.

2. Yogurt Parfait

- **Ingredients:**
    - 1 cup Greek yogurt

- ½ cup smooth oats, cooked
- 1 tablespoon honey
- ¼ cup canned peaches, diced

- **Instructions:**

1. In a portable container, layer the Greek yogurt, cooked oats, and peaches.

2. Drizzle with honey and seal with a lid.

3. Refrigerate until ready to eat.

- **Benefits:**
    - This parfait is rich in protein and fiber, making it a convenient and satisfying breakfast option.

3. Overnight Chia Pudding

- **Ingredients:**
    - 2 tablespoons chia seeds
    - 1 cup lactose-free milk
    - 1 tablespoon honey
    - ¼ teaspoon vanilla extract

- **Instructions:**

1. In a jar or container, combine the chia seeds, lactose-free milk, honey, and vanilla extract.

2. Stir well and refrigerate overnight.

3. In the morning, give it a stir and enjoy.

- **Benefits:**
    - Chia pudding is easy to prepare in advance and provides a nutrient-dense start to your day with omega-3s and fiber.

4. Smoothie Packets

- **Ingredients:**
    - 1 banana
    - ½ cup berries (strawberries, blueberries, or raspberries)
    - ¼ cup spinach (optional)
    - 1 tablespoon honey
- **Instructions:**

1. In a resealable freezer bag, combine the banana, berries, and spinach.

2. Freeze until ready to use.

3. In the morning, blend the contents with a cup of lactose-free milk and honey.

- **Benefits:**

- These smoothie packets make breakfast preparation quick and easy, while providing a nutritious start to your day.

5. Soft Muffins

- **Ingredients:**
    - 1 cup all-purpose flour
    - 1 teaspoon baking powder
    - 1/2 teaspoon baking soda
    - 1/4 cup honey
    - 1 egg
    - 1/2 cup lactose-free yogurt
    - 1/4 cup vegetable oil
    - 1 ripe banana, mashed
- **Instructions:**

1. Preheat the oven to 350°F (175°C).

2. In a bowl, mix the flour, baking powder, and baking soda.

3. In another bowl, whisk together the honey, egg, yogurt, oil, and mashed banana.

4. Combine the wet and dry ingredients until just mixed.

5. Pour the batter into muffin tins and bake for 15-20 minutes.

6. Allow to cool before storing in an airtight container.

- **Benefits:**
    - These muffins are soft, easy to digest, and can be made in advance, making them perfect for a quick grab-and-go breakfast.

6. Apple and Cheese Snack Box

- **Ingredients:**
    - 1 apple, peeled and sliced
    - 1/4 cup lactose-free cheese, cubed
    - 1 handful of soft crackers
- **Instructions:**

1. Pack the apple slices, cheese cubes, and crackers in a portable container.

2. Keep refrigerated until ready to eat.

- **Benefits:**
    - This snack box is balanced, offering a mix of fiber, protein, and carbohydrates in a portable format.

7. Egg Muffins

- **Ingredients:**
    - 4 eggs
    - 1/2 cup diced vegetables (bell peppers, spinach, etc.)
    - 1/4 cup lactose-free cheese, shredded
    - A pinch of salt and pepper
- **Instructions:**

1. Preheat the oven to 350°F (175°C).
2. Grease a muffin tin and evenly distribute the vegetables and cheese.
3. Whisk the eggs with salt and pepper, then pour into the muffin tin.
4. Bake for 15-20 minutes, or until the eggs are set.
5. Allow to cool before storing in the refrigerator.

- **Benefits:**
    - Egg muffins are protein-packed, easy to prepare in advance, and can be eaten on the go.

8. Cottage Cheese and Pineapple Bowl

- **Ingredients:**
    - 1 cup cottage cheese

- 1/2 cup canned pineapple, diced
- 1 tablespoon honey

- **Instructions:**

1. In a portable container, mix the cottage cheese, pineapple, and honey.
2. Seal with a lid and refrigerate until ready to eat.

- **Benefits:**
  - This combination is high in protein and gentle on the digestive system, perfect for a light and refreshing breakfast.

9. Avocado and Hummus Wrap

- **Ingredients:**
  - 1 soft whole-wheat tortilla
  - 1/2 avocado, mashed
  - 2 tablespoons hummus

- **Instructions:**

1. Spread the hummus on the tortilla.
2. Add the mashed avocado and spread evenly.
3. Roll up the tortilla and slice in half.

- **Benefits:**

- This wrap is rich in healthy fats and fiber, making it a satisfying and portable breakfast option.

10. Peanut Butter and Banana Rice Cake

- **Ingredients:**
  - 1 rice cake
  - 2 tablespoons peanut butter
  - 1 banana, sliced
- **Instructions:**
1. Spread peanut butter on the rice cake.
2. Top with banana slices.
3. Pack in a portable container and enjoy on the go.
- **Benefits:**
  - This simple snack is rich in protein and carbohydrates, providing quick energy and easy digestion.

Chapter 5: Lunch Ideas for Sustained Energy

10 Wholesome Soups and Broths

Soups and broths are excellent options for lunch, especially during recovery. They are easy to digest, hydrating, and can be packed with nutrients that support healing. Here are 10 wholesome recipes to keep you nourished and satisfied.

1. Chicken and Vegetable Broth

- **Ingredients:**
    - 1 chicken breast, cooked and shredded
    - 1 carrot, diced
    - 1 celery stalk, diced
    - 1 small potato, diced
    - 4 cups low-sodium chicken broth
    - 1 bay leaf
    - Salt and pepper to taste
- **Instructions:**

1. In a pot, combine the chicken broth, carrot, celery, potato, and bay leaf.

2. Bring to a boil, then reduce the heat and simmer until the vegetables are tender.

3. Add the shredded chicken and cook for another 5 minutes.

4. Season with salt and pepper before serving.

- **Benefits:**
  - This broth is soothing, protein-rich, and full of essential vitamins and minerals, perfect for a light but nourishing lunch.

2. Creamy Carrot and Ginger Soup

- **Ingredients:**
  - 4 large carrots, peeled and chopped
  - 1 small onion, chopped
  - 1 tablespoon fresh ginger, grated
  - 4 cups low-sodium vegetable broth
  - 1/2 cup lactose-free cream
  - 1 tablespoon olive oil
  - Salt and pepper to taste

- **Instructions:**

1. Heat olive oil in a large pot and sauté the onion and ginger until fragrant.

2. Add the carrots and vegetable broth, then bring to a boil.

3. Reduce heat and simmer until the carrots are soft.

4. Use an immersion blender to puree the soup until smooth.

5. Stir in the cream and season with salt and pepper.

- **Benefits:**
  - This creamy soup is gentle on the stomach, with anti-inflammatory properties from the ginger to support recovery.

3. Butternut Squash Soup

- **Ingredients:**
  - 1 medium butternut squash, peeled and cubed
  - 1 small onion, chopped
  - 2 cloves garlic, minced
  - 4 cups low-sodium chicken broth
  - 1/2 cup lactose-free milk
  - 1 tablespoon olive oil
  - Salt and pepper to taste
- **Instructions:**

1. Heat olive oil in a large pot and sauté the onion and garlic until soft.

2. Add the butternut squash and chicken broth, then bring to a boil.

3. Reduce the heat and simmer until the squash is tender.

4. Puree the soup with an immersion blender until smooth.

5. Stir in the milk and season with salt and pepper.

- **Benefits:**
    - Packed with vitamins A and C, this soup is both nourishing and delicious, with a creamy texture that's easy on the digestive system.

4. Chicken Noodle Soup

- **Ingredients:**
    - 1 chicken breast, cooked and shredded
    - 1 cup egg noodles
    - 1 carrot, sliced
    - 1 celery stalk, sliced
    - 4 cups low-sodium chicken broth
    - 1 bay leaf

- Salt and pepper to taste

- **Instructions:**

1. In a pot, bring the chicken broth, carrot, celery, and bay leaf to a boil.

2. Add the egg noodles and cook until tender.

3. Stir in the shredded chicken and cook for another 5 minutes.

4. Season with salt and pepper before serving.

- **Benefits:**
  - This classic comfort soup is easy to digest and provides a balanced mix of protein and carbohydrates for sustained energy.

5. Potato Leek Soup

- **Ingredients:**
  - 4 medium potatoes, peeled and diced
  - 2 leeks, white part only, sliced
  - 4 cups low-sodium vegetable broth
  - 1/2 cup lactose-free cream
  - 1 tablespoon olive oil
  - Salt and pepper to taste

- **Instructions:**

1. In a large pot, heat the olive oil and sauté the leeks until soft.

2. Add the potatoes and vegetable broth, then bring to a boil.

3. Reduce the heat and simmer until the potatoes are tender.

4. Puree the soup with an immersion blender until smooth.

5. Stir in the cream and season with salt and pepper.

- **Benefits:**
    - This hearty soup is creamy and satisfying, with the added benefit of being gentle on your digestive system.

6. Tomato Basil Soup

- **Ingredients:**
    - 4 large tomatoes, peeled and chopped
    - 1 small onion, chopped
    - 2 cloves garlic, minced
    - 4 cups low-sodium vegetable broth
    - 1/2 cup lactose-free cream
    - 1 tablespoon olive oil
    - 1/4 cup fresh basil leaves

- Salt and pepper to taste

- **Instructions:**

1. Heat olive oil in a large pot and sauté the onion and garlic until soft.

2. Add the tomatoes and vegetable broth, then bring to a boil.

3. Reduce the heat and simmer until the tomatoes are soft.

4. Puree the soup with an immersion blender until smooth.

5. Stir in the cream and basil, then season with salt and pepper.

- **Benefits:**
    - This vibrant soup is rich in antioxidants and offers a refreshing taste of basil, making it both nourishing and delicious.

7. Miso Soup with Tofu

- **Ingredients:**
    - 4 cups water
    - 1/4 cup miso paste
    - 1/2 block tofu, cubed
    - 1 green onion, sliced

- 1 sheet seaweed, cut into strips
- **Instructions:**

1. In a pot, bring the water to a boil, then reduce the heat to low.
2. Whisk in the miso paste until dissolved.
3. Add the tofu and seaweed, and cook for 5 minutes.
4. Garnish with green onion before serving.

- **Benefits:**
  - Miso soup is light yet packed with umami flavor, offering a soothing and easy-to-digest option that's rich in probiotics.

8. Beef and Barley Soup

- **Ingredients:**
  - 1/2 pound lean beef, cubed
  - 1/2 cup barley
  - 1 carrot, diced
  - 1 celery stalk, diced
  - 4 cups low-sodium beef broth
  - 1 bay leaf
  - Salt and pepper to taste
- **Instructions:**

1. In a pot, bring the beef broth, carrot, celery, and bay leaf to a boil.

2. Add the beef and barley, then reduce the heat and simmer until tender.

3. Season with salt and pepper before serving.

- **Benefits:**
    - This hearty soup is full of protein and fiber, providing sustained energy throughout the day.

9. Lentil Soup

- **Ingredients:**
    - 1 cup red lentils, rinsed
    - 1 small onion, chopped
    - 2 cloves garlic, minced
    - 1 carrot, diced
    - 4 cups low-sodium vegetable broth
    - 1 teaspoon cumin
    - 1 tablespoon olive oil
    - Salt and pepper to taste
- **Instructions:**

1. Heat olive oil in a large pot and sauté the onion, garlic, and carrot until soft.

2. Add the lentils, vegetable broth, and cumin, then bring to a boil.

3. Reduce the heat and simmer until the lentils are tender.

4. Season with salt and pepper before serving.

- **Benefits:**
  - This lentil soup is rich in protein and fiber, offering a filling and nutritious meal that's easy on the digestive system.

10. Pumpkin Soup

- **Ingredients:**
  - 2 cups pumpkin puree
  - 1 small onion, chopped
  - 2 cloves garlic, minced
  - 4 cups low-sodium chicken broth
  - 1/2 cup lactose-free cream
  - 1 tablespoon olive oil
  - Salt and pepper to taste
- **Instructions:**

1. Heat olive oil in a large pot and sauté the onion and garlic until soft.

2. Add the pumpkin puree and chicken broth, then bring to a boil.

3. Reduce the heat and simmer for 10 minutes.

4. Puree the soup with an immersion blender until smooth.

5. Stir in the cream and season with salt and pepper.

- **Benefits:**
    - This creamy pumpkin soup is rich in vitamins A and C, supporting overall health and recovery while being easy on digestion.

10 Protein-Packed Salads and Wraps

Protein is essential for recovery and sustained energy, especially during lunchtime. These salads and wraps are designed to be both delicious and easy to digest, offering a variety of flavors and textures to keep your meals interesting.

1. Chicken Caesar Salad

- **Ingredients:**
    - 1 cup romaine lettuce, chopped

- 1/2 cup cooked chicken breast, sliced
- 2 tablespoons lactose-free Caesar dressing
- 1 tablespoon grated Parmesan cheese
- A handful of croutons

- **Instructions:**

1. In a bowl, combine the lettuce, chicken, and dressing.
2. Toss until well coated.
3. Top with Parmesan cheese and croutons before serving.

- **Benefits:**
  - This classic salad is protein-rich and full of flavor, offering a satisfying and nutritious lunch option.

2. Turkey and Avocado Wrap

- **Ingredients:**
  - 1 soft whole-wheat tortilla
  - 2 slices of turkey breast
  - 1/2 avocado, sliced
  - 1/4 cup spinach leaves

- 1 tablespoon mayonnaise

- **Instructions:**

1. Spread mayonnaise on the tortilla.
2. Layer the turkey, avocado, and spinach on top.
3. Roll up the tortilla and slice in half.

- **Benefits:**
    - This wrap is rich in healthy fats and lean protein, making it a nourishing and easy-to-eat lunch option.

3. Quinoa and Grilled Vegetable Salad

- **Ingredients:**
    - 1/2 cup cooked quinoa
    - 1/4 cup grilled zucchini, diced
    - 1/4 cup grilled bell pepper, diced
    - 1/4 cup grilled eggplant, diced
    - 1 tablespoon olive oil
    - 1 tablespoon balsamic vinegar
    - Salt and pepper to taste
- **Instructions:**

1. In a bowl, combine the cooked quinoa and grilled vegetables.

2. Drizzle with olive oil and balsamic vinegar.

3. Season with salt and pepper before serving.

- **Benefits:**
    - Quinoa is a complete protein, providing all essential amino acids, while the grilled vegetables add fiber and flavor.

4. Egg Salad Lettuce Wraps

- **Ingredients:**
    - 2 hard-boiled eggs, chopped
    - 1 tablespoon mayonnaise
    - 1 teaspoon Dijon mustard
    - 1 celery stalk, finely chopped
    - 4 large lettuce leaves
- **Instructions:**

1. In a bowl, mix the chopped eggs, mayonnaise, mustard, and celery.

2. Spoon the egg salad onto the lettuce leaves.

3. Roll up the lettuce wraps and serve.

- **Benefits:**
    - These wraps are high in protein and low in carbs, making them light yet filling.

5. Tuna Salad Sandwich

- **Ingredients:**
    - 1 can of tuna, drained
    - 2 tablespoons mayonnaise
    - 1 celery stalk, chopped
    - 1 tablespoon lemon juice
    - 2 slices of soft whole-wheat bread
- **Instructions:**

1. In a bowl, mix the tuna, mayonnaise, celery, and lemon juice.
2. Spread the tuna salad evenly over one slice of bread.
3. Top with the other slice and cut in half.

- **Benefits:**
    - Tuna is an excellent source of lean protein and omega-3 fatty acids, promoting heart health and muscle recovery.

6. Greek Chicken Salad

- **Ingredients:**
    - 1 cup romaine lettuce, chopped
    - 1/2 cup cooked chicken breast, diced

- 1/4 cup cucumber, diced
- 1/4 cup cherry tomatoes, halved
- 1/4 cup crumbled feta cheese
- 2 tablespoons olive oil
- 1 tablespoon lemon juice

- **Instructions:**

1. In a large bowl, combine the lettuce, chicken, cucumber, tomatoes, and feta.

2. Drizzle with olive oil and lemon juice.

3. Toss well and serve.

- **Benefits:**
  - This salad is packed with protein and healthy fats, offering a refreshing and satisfying lunch.

7. Hummus and Veggie Wrap

- **Ingredients:**
  - 1 soft whole-wheat tortilla
  - 3 tablespoons hummus
  - 1/4 cup shredded carrots
  - 1/4 cup cucumber, sliced
  - 1/4 cup bell pepper, sliced

- **Instructions:**
1. Spread the hummus evenly over the tortilla.
2. Layer the vegetables on top.
3. Roll up the tortilla and slice in half.
- **Benefits:**
    o This wrap is rich in fiber and plant-based protein, making it a nutritious and easy-to-digest option.

8. Shrimp and Avocado Salad

- **Ingredients:**
    o 1/2 cup cooked shrimp, peeled and deveined
    o 1/2 avocado, sliced
    o 1 cup mixed greens
    o 1 tablespoon olive oil
    o 1 tablespoon lime juice
    o Salt and pepper to taste
- **Instructions:**
1. In a large bowl, combine the mixed greens, shrimp, and avocado.
2. Drizzle with olive oil and lime juice.
3. Toss gently and season with salt and pepper.

- **Benefits:**
  - This salad is high in healthy fats and protein, offering a light yet satisfying meal.

9. Turkey and Cheese Wrap

- **Ingredients:**
  - 1 soft whole-wheat tortilla
  - 2 slices of turkey breast
  - 1 slice lactose-free cheese
  - 1/4 cup spinach leaves
  - 1 tablespoon mayonnaise
- **Instructions:**

1. Spread mayonnaise on the tortilla.
2. Layer the turkey, cheese, and spinach on top.
3. Roll up the tortilla and slice in half.

- **Benefits:**
  - This wrap is balanced in protein and healthy fats, making it an ideal lunch for sustained energy.

10. Chicken and Avocado Salad

- **Ingredients:**
  - 1 cup mixed greens

- o 1/2 avocado, sliced
- o 1/2 cup cooked chicken breast, diced
- o 1 tablespoon olive oil
- o 1 tablespoon balsamic vinegar
- o Salt and pepper to taste

- **Instructions:**

1. In a large bowl, combine the mixed greens, avocado, and chicken.

2. Drizzle with olive oil and balsamic vinegar.

3. Toss gently and season with salt and pepper.

- **Benefits:**
  - o This salad is rich in protein and healthy fats, making it a nourishing and easy-to-digest option for lunch.

10 Nutrient-Dense Sandwiches and Toasts

Sandwiches and toasts are versatile and satisfying lunch options that can be tailored to your dietary needs. These recipes focus on nutrient density while being gentle on the digestive system.

1. Turkey and Avocado Sandwich

- **Ingredients:**

- 2 slices of soft whole-wheat bread
- 2 slices of turkey breast
- 1/2 avocado, mashed
- 1 slice lactose-free cheese

- **Instructions:**

1. Spread the mashed avocado on one slice of bread.
2. Layer the turkey and cheese on top.
3. Top with the other slice of bread and cut in half.

- **Benefits:**
  - This sandwich is packed with lean protein and healthy fats, making it both delicious and nourishing.

2. Egg and Spinach Toast

- **Ingredients:**
  - 1 slice of soft whole-wheat bread, toasted
  - 1 hard-boiled egg, sliced
  - 1/4 cup sautéed spinach
  - Salt and pepper to taste

- **Instructions:**

1. Layer the sliced egg and sautéed spinach on the toast.

2. Season with salt and pepper before serving.
- **Benefits:**
    - This toast is high in protein and iron, supporting energy levels and overall health.

3. Hummus and Veggie Sandwich

- **Ingredients:**
    - 2 slices of soft whole-wheat bread
    - 3 tablespoons hummus
    - 1/4 cup shredded carrots
    - 1/4 cup cucumber, sliced
    - 1/4 cup bell pepper, sliced
- **Instructions:**
1. Spread the hummus on one slice of bread.
2. Layer the vegetables on top.
3. Top with the other slice of bread and cut in half.
- **Benefits:**
    - This sandwich is rich in fiber and plant-based protein, making it a nutritious and easy-to-digest option.

4. Chicken and Pesto Toast

- **Ingredients:**

- 1 slice of soft whole-wheat bread, toasted
- 1/2 cup cooked chicken breast, shredded
- 2 tablespoons pesto sauce

- **Instructions:**

1. Spread the pesto sauce on the toast.
2. Top with the shredded chicken and serve.

- **Benefits:**
  - This toast is high in protein and flavor, offering a satisfying and quick lunch option.

5. Peanut Butter and Banana Sandwich

- **Ingredients:**
  - 2 slices of soft whole-wheat bread
  - 2 tablespoons peanut butter
  - 1 banana, sliced

- **Instructions:**

1. Spread peanut butter on one slice of bread.
2. Layer the banana slices on top.
3. Top with the other slice of bread and cut in half.

- **Benefits:**

- This sandwich is rich in protein and carbohydrates, providing quick energy and easy digestion.

6. Avocado and Tomato Toast

- **Ingredients:**
  - 1 slice of soft whole-wheat bread, toasted
  - 1/2 avocado, mashed
  - 1 small tomato, sliced
  - Salt and pepper to taste
- **Instructions:**
1. Spread the mashed avocado on the toast.
2. Layer the tomato slices on top.
3. Season with salt and pepper before serving.
- **Benefits:**
  - This toast is rich in healthy fats and antioxidants, making it a nourishing and satisfying option.

7. Tuna and Cucumber Sandwich

- **Ingredients:**
  - 2 slices of soft whole-wheat bread
  - 1 can of tuna, drained

- o 1 tablespoon mayonnaise
- o 1/4 cup cucumber, sliced
- **Instructions:**
1. Mix the tuna with mayonnaise in a bowl.
2. Spread the tuna mixture on one slice of bread.
3. Layer the cucumber slices on top.
4. Top with the other slice of bread and cut in half.
- **Benefits:**
  - o This sandwich is high in protein and omega-3 fatty acids, promoting heart health and muscle recovery.

8. Turkey and Cranberry Sandwich

- **Ingredients:**
  - o 2 slices of soft whole-wheat bread
  - o 2 slices of turkey breast
  - o 2 tablespoons cranberry sauce
  - o 1 slice lactose-free cheese
- **Instructions:**
1. Spread the cranberry sauce on one slice of bread.
2. Layer the turkey and cheese on top.

3. Top with the other slice of bread and cut in half.
- **Benefits:**
  - This sandwich combines lean protein with antioxidants, offering a flavorful and healthy lunch option.

9. Egg Salad Sandwich

- **Ingredients:**
  - 2 hard-boiled eggs, chopped
  - 2 tablespoons mayonnaise
  - 1 celery stalk, chopped
  - 2 slices of soft whole-wheat bread
- **Instructions:**

1. In a bowl, mix the chopped eggs, mayonnaise, and celery.

2. Spread the egg salad on one slice of bread.

3. Top with the other slice of bread and cut in half.

- **Benefits:**
  - This sandwich is high in protein and easy to digest, making it a satisfying and gentle lunch option.

10. Salmon and Avocado Toast

- **Ingredients:**
    - 1 slice of soft whole-wheat bread, toasted
    - 1/2 avocado, sliced
    - 1/4 cup cooked salmon, flaked
    - 1 tablespoon lemon juice
- **Instructions:**

1. Layer the avocado slices on the toast.
2. Top with flaked salmon and drizzle with lemon juice.

- **Benefits:**
    - This toast is rich in omega-3 fatty acids and healthy fats, making it a nourishing and flavorful choice.

10 Portable Lunchbox Favorites

When you're on the go, having a selection of portable, nutrient-dense meals is essential. These recipes are designed to be easy to pack, store, and enjoy wherever your day takes you.

1. Chicken and Rice Salad

- **Ingredients:**

- 1/2 cup cooked brown rice
- 1/2 cup cooked chicken breast, diced
- 1/4 cup diced cucumber
- 1/4 cup cherry tomatoes, halved
- 1 tablespoon olive oil
- 1 tablespoon lemon juice
- Salt and pepper to taste

- **Instructions:**

1. In a large bowl, combine the rice, chicken, cucumber, and cherry tomatoes.
2. Drizzle with olive oil and lemon juice.
3. Season with salt and pepper, then toss to mix.
4. Pack in a portable container for easy transport.

- **Benefits:**
    - This salad is balanced in protein and carbohydrates, providing sustained energy throughout the day.

2. Turkey and Cheese Roll-Ups

- **Ingredients:**
    - 4 slices of turkey breast
    - 2 slices lactose-free cheese

- 1/4 cup spinach leaves
- 1 tablespoon mustard or mayonnaise

- **Instructions:**

1. Lay out the turkey slices and spread with mustard or mayonnaise.

2. Place a slice of cheese and some spinach leaves on top of each turkey slice.

3. Roll up the turkey slices and secure with toothpicks if needed.

4. Pack in a container for a quick and portable meal.

- **Benefits:**
  - These roll-ups are high in protein and low in carbs, making them a light and satisfying option.

3. Quinoa and Veggie Mason Jar Salad

- **Ingredients:**
  - 1/2 cup cooked quinoa
  - 1/4 cup diced bell peppers
  - 1/4 cup diced cucumber
  - 1/4 cup cherry tomatoes, halved
  - 2 tablespoons hummus

- 1 tablespoon lemon juice
- Salt and pepper to taste

- **Instructions:**

1. In a mason jar, layer the quinoa, bell peppers, cucumber, and cherry tomatoes.

2. Top with hummus and lemon juice.

3. Season with salt and pepper.

4. Seal the jar and store in the fridge until ready to eat.

- **Benefits:**
  - This salad is nutrient-dense and easy to carry, making it perfect for meal prep and on-the-go eating.

4. Hummus and Veggie Bento Box

- **Ingredients:**
  - 1/4 cup hummus
  - 1/4 cup baby carrots
  - 1/4 cup cucumber slices
  - 1/4 cup cherry tomatoes
  - 1/4 cup whole-wheat pita bread, cut into triangles

- **Instructions:**

1. Pack the hummus in a small container.

2. Arrange the vegetables and pita triangles in a bento box.

3. Add the hummus container to the box for dipping.

- **Benefits:**
    - This bento box is rich in fiber and plant-based protein, making it a healthy and convenient lunch option.

5. Chicken and Avocado Sushi Rolls

- **Ingredients:**
    - 1/2 cup cooked sushi rice
    - 1/4 cup cooked chicken breast, shredded
    - 1/4 avocado, sliced
    - 1 sheet of nori (seaweed)
    - 1 tablespoon soy sauce (optional)

- **Instructions:**

1. Spread the sushi rice evenly over the nori sheet.

2. Layer the shredded chicken and avocado slices on top.

3. Roll up the nori tightly, then slice into bite-sized pieces.

4. Pack in a container with soy sauce for dipping if desired.

- **Benefits:**
  - These sushi rolls are light, flavorful, and easy to pack, offering a nutritious lunch option that's perfect for on-the-go.

6. Pasta Salad with Pesto and Veggies

- **Ingredients:**
  - 1/2 cup cooked whole-wheat pasta
  - 1/4 cup diced bell peppers
  - 1/4 cup cherry tomatoes, halved
  - 1/4 cup diced cucumber
  - 2 tablespoons pesto sauce
- **Instructions:**

1. In a large bowl, mix the cooked pasta, bell peppers, cherry tomatoes, and cucumber.

2. Add the pesto sauce and toss to coat.

3. Pack in a container and refrigerate until ready to eat.

- **Benefits:**

- This pasta salad is balanced in carbs and healthy fats, making it a satisfying and easy-to-digest meal.

7. Protein-Packed Snack Box

- **Ingredients:**
  - 1/4 cup cubed cheese
  - 1/4 cup sliced turkey breast
  - 1/4 cup almonds
  - 1/4 cup baby carrots
- **Instructions:**

1. Arrange the cheese, turkey slices, almonds, and baby carrots in a snack box.
2. Seal the box and keep it chilled until ready to eat.

- **Benefits:**
  - This snack box is high in protein and healthy fats, providing a quick and balanced meal or snack on the go.

8. Fruit and Nut Energy Bites

- **Ingredients:**
  - 1/2 cup rolled oats
  - 1/4 cup almond butter

- 1/4 cup honey
- 1/4 cup dried cranberries
- 1/4 cup chopped nuts

- **Instructions:**

1. In a bowl, mix the rolled oats, almond butter, honey, dried cranberries, and chopped nuts.

2. Roll the mixture into small balls.

3. Pack in a container and refrigerate until ready to eat.

- **Benefits:**
  - These energy bites are packed with fiber and healthy fats, making them a perfect portable snack or small meal.

9. Greek Yogurt and Berry Parfait

- **Ingredients:**
  - 1/2 cup lactose-free Greek yogurt
  - 1/4 cup mixed berries
  - 1 tablespoon honey
  - 1 tablespoon granola (optional)
- **Instructions:**

1. Layer the Greek yogurt and mixed berries in a small container.

2. Drizzle with honey and sprinkle granola on top if desired.

3. Seal the container and store in the fridge until ready to eat.

- **Benefits:**
    - This parfait is rich in protein and antioxidants, offering a refreshing and healthy meal or snack option.

10. Vegetable and Cheese Muffins

- **Ingredients:**
    - 1/2 cup grated zucchini
    - 1/2 cup grated carrots
    - 1/4 cup shredded lactose-free cheese
    - 2 eggs
    - 1/4 cup whole-wheat flour
    - Salt and pepper to taste
- **Instructions:**

1. Preheat the oven to 350°F (175°C) and grease a muffin tin.

2. In a bowl, mix the grated zucchini, carrots, cheese, eggs, and flour.

3. Season with salt and pepper.

4. Spoon the mixture into the muffin tin and bake for 20-25 minutes, or until golden brown.

5. Let the muffins cool before packing them in a container.

- **Benefits:**
    - These muffins are nutrient-dense and easy to carry, making them a great option for a portable and filling lunch.

Chapter 6: Dinner Recipes for Comfort and Healing

Dinner is often the most anticipated meal of the day, and during your recovery, it's important to focus on comfort, nutrition, and easy digestion. This chapter provides a variety of dinner recipes that are gentle on your digestive system while being packed with essential nutrients to support healing and restore your energy.

Nourishing One-Pot Meals

One-pot meals are perfect for minimizing cleanup while delivering all the essential nutrients you need. These recipes are designed to be simple, hearty, and comforting.

1. Chicken and Vegetable Stew

- **Ingredients:**
    - 2 chicken breasts, diced
    - 1 cup carrots, diced
    - 1 cup potatoes, diced
    - 1 cup celery, sliced
    - 1 onion, chopped
    - 4 cups low-sodium chicken broth
    - 1 tablespoon olive oil

- o 1 teaspoon thyme
- o Salt and pepper to taste

- **Instructions:**

1. In a large pot, heat the olive oil over medium heat. Add the onion and sauté until softened.

2. Add the chicken and cook until browned on all sides.

3. Add the carrots, potatoes, celery, thyme, salt, and pepper. Pour in the chicken broth.

4. Bring to a boil, then reduce the heat and let simmer for 30-40 minutes, or until the vegetables are tender.

5. Serve warm for a comforting, nutrient-rich meal.

- **Benefits:**
  - o This stew is high in protein and packed with vegetables, making it a nourishing and easy-to-digest dinner option.

2. Beef and Barley Soup

- **Ingredients:**
  - o 1/2 pound lean beef stew meat, cubed
  - o 1/2 cup barley
  - o 1 cup carrots, sliced
  - o 1 cup celery, sliced

- 1 onion, chopped
- 4 cups low-sodium beef broth
- 1 tablespoon olive oil
- 1 teaspoon thyme
- Salt and pepper to taste

- **Instructions:**

1. In a large pot, heat the olive oil over medium heat. Add the onion and cook until softened.

2. Add the beef and cook until browned on all sides.

3. Add the carrots, celery, barley, thyme, salt, and pepper. Pour in the beef broth.

4. Bring to a boil, then reduce the heat and simmer for 45-60 minutes, or until the barley is tender.

5. Serve hot for a hearty and filling meal.

- **Benefits:**
  - This one-pot meal provides a balance of protein, fiber, and complex carbohydrates, making it ideal for a soothing dinner.

3. Turkey and Sweet Potato Chili

- **Ingredients:**
  - 1 pound ground turkey

- 2 cups sweet potatoes, diced
- 1 onion, chopped
- 2 cloves garlic, minced
- 1 can (15 oz) low-sodium diced tomatoes
- 1 can (15 oz) kidney beans, drained and rinsed
- 2 cups low-sodium chicken broth
- 1 tablespoon chili powder
- 1 teaspoon cumin
- Salt and pepper to taste

- **Instructions:**

1. In a large pot, cook the ground turkey over medium heat until browned. Drain excess fat.

2. Add the onion and garlic, cooking until softened.

3. Add the sweet potatoes, diced tomatoes, kidney beans, chicken broth, chili powder, cumin, salt, and pepper.

4. Bring to a boil, then reduce the heat and simmer for 30-40 minutes, or until the sweet potatoes are tender.

5. Serve warm for a comforting, protein-rich meal.

- **Benefits:**

- This chili is rich in lean protein and complex carbs, providing a hearty and satisfying dinner option that's gentle on your digestive system.

4. **Lentil and Vegetable Curry**

- **Ingredients:**
    - 1 cup lentils, rinsed
    - 1 cup carrots, diced
    - 1 cup potatoes, diced
    - 1 onion, chopped
    - 2 cloves garlic, minced
    - 1 can (15 oz) coconut milk
    - 2 cups vegetable broth
    - 1 tablespoon curry powder
    - 1 teaspoon turmeric
    - Salt and pepper to taste
- **Instructions:**

1. In a large pot, sauté the onion and garlic in a bit of olive oil until softened.

2. Add the carrots, potatoes, lentils, curry powder, turmeric, salt, and pepper. Stir to combine.

3. Pour in the coconut milk and vegetable broth, bringing the mixture to a boil.

4. Reduce the heat and simmer for 30-40 minutes, or until the lentils and vegetables are tender.

5. Serve warm with a side of soft bread or rice.

- **Benefits:**
  - This curry is rich in plant-based protein and anti-inflammatory spices, making it a flavorful and nourishing option for dinner.

5. Creamy Chicken and Rice Casserole

- **Ingredients:**
  - 2 cups cooked brown rice
  - 1 cup cooked chicken breast, shredded
  - 1 cup broccoli florets, steamed
  - 1 cup lactose-free cream
  - 1/2 cup lactose-free cheese, shredded
  - 1/4 cup breadcrumbs
  - 1 tablespoon olive oil
  - Salt and pepper to taste
- **Instructions:**

1. Preheat the oven to 350°F (175°C).

2.   In a large bowl, combine the cooked rice, chicken, broccoli, cream, salt, and pepper.

3.   Transfer the mixture to a greased baking dish. Top with shredded cheese and breadcrumbs.

4.   Drizzle with olive oil and bake for 25-30 minutes, or until the top is golden and bubbly.

5.   Serve hot for a comforting and filling meal.

- **Benefits:**
    - This casserole is high in protein and calcium, making it a hearty and nourishing dinner that's easy to prepare.

Flavorful Pasta and Rice Dishes

Pasta and rice dishes are comforting staples that can be easily adapted to suit your dietary needs during recovery. These recipes offer a balance of flavor and nutrition, making them perfect for a satisfying dinner.

1. Creamy Chicken Alfredo

- **Ingredients:**
    - 8 oz fettuccine pasta (softened)

- 1 cup cooked chicken breast, sliced
- 1/2 cup lactose-free cream
- 1/2 cup lactose-free parmesan cheese, grated
- 2 cloves garlic, minced
- 2 tablespoons olive oil
- Salt and pepper to taste

- **Instructions:**

1. Cook the fettuccine according to package instructions. Drain and set aside.

2. In a large pan, heat the olive oil over medium heat and sauté the garlic until fragrant.

3. Add the cooked chicken and stir until heated through.

4. Pour in the lactose-free cream and bring to a simmer.

5. Stir in the grated parmesan cheese until the sauce is smooth and creamy.

6. Toss the cooked fettuccine in the sauce and season with salt and pepper.

7. Serve hot with an extra sprinkle of parmesan cheese.

- **Benefits:**

- This dish is rich in protein and calcium, providing a creamy and comforting meal that's easy on your stomach.

2. Vegetable Risotto

- **Ingredients:**
  - 1 cup Arborio rice
  - 1/2 cup diced carrots
  - 1/2 cup diced zucchini
  - 1/2 cup green peas
  - 4 cups low-sodium vegetable broth, warmed
  - 1/4 cup lactose-free parmesan cheese, grated
  - 2 tablespoons olive oil
  - 1 small onion, finely chopped
  - Salt and pepper to taste
- **Instructions:**

1. In a large pan, heat the olive oil over medium heat and sauté the onion until softened.

2. Add the Arborio rice and stir for 2-3 minutes until the rice is lightly toasted.

3. Gradually add the warm vegetable broth, one ladleful at a time, stirring constantly until the liquid is absorbed before adding more.

4. After about 15 minutes, stir in the diced carrots, zucchini, and green peas.

5. Continue cooking and stirring until the rice is creamy and tender, about 20-25 minutes in total.

6. Stir in the grated parmesan cheese and season with salt and pepper.

7. Serve warm for a creamy and nourishing meal.

- **Benefits:**
    - This risotto is packed with vegetables and provides a good balance of carbohydrates and protein, making it a satisfying and gentle option.

3. Lemon Garlic Shrimp Pasta

- **Ingredients:**
    - 8 oz spaghetti pasta (softened)
    - 1/2 pound shrimp, peeled and deveined
    - 3 cloves garlic, minced
    - 1/4 cup olive oil
    - 1/4 cup fresh lemon juice
    - 2 tablespoons fresh parsley, chopped
    - Salt and pepper to taste
- **Instructions:**

1. Cook the spaghetti according to package instructions. Drain and set aside.

2. In a large pan, heat the olive oil over medium heat and sauté the garlic until fragrant.

3. Add the shrimp and cook until pink and opaque, about 3-4 minutes.

4. Stir in the lemon juice and season with salt and pepper.

5. Toss the cooked spaghetti in the sauce and sprinkle with fresh parsley.

6. Serve warm with a drizzle of extra olive oil.

- **Benefits:**
    - This pasta dish is rich in protein and healthy fats, offering a light and flavorful meal that's easy to digest.

4. Mushroom and Spinach Risotto

- **Ingredients:**
    - 1 cup Arborio rice
    - 1 cup mushrooms, sliced
    - 1 cup baby spinach
    - 4 cups low-sodium vegetable broth, warmed
    - 1/4 cup lactose-free parmesan cheese, grated

- 2 tablespoons olive oil
- 1 small onion, finely chopped
- 2 cloves garlic, minced
- Salt and pepper to taste

- **Instructions:**

1. In a large pan, heat the olive oil over medium heat and sauté the onion and garlic until softened.

2. Add the mushrooms and cook until they release their moisture and are browned.

3. Add the Arborio rice and stir for 2-3 minutes until the rice is lightly toasted.

4. Gradually add the warm vegetable broth, one ladleful at a time, stirring constantly until the liquid is absorbed before adding more.

5. After about 15 minutes, stir in the baby spinach and continue cooking until the rice is creamy and tender, about 20-25 minutes in total.

6. Stir in the grated parmesan cheese and season with salt and pepper.

7. Serve warm for a comforting and nutrient-rich meal.

- **Benefits:**

- This risotto is a great source of fiber, protein, and antioxidants, making it a nourishing option for dinner.

5. Chicken and Broccoli Stir-Fry with Rice

- **Ingredients:**
    - 1 cup cooked brown rice
    - 1 chicken breast, sliced thinly
    - 1 cup broccoli florets
    - 2 tablespoons soy sauce (low sodium)
    - 1 tablespoon olive oil
    - 2 cloves garlic, minced
    - 1 teaspoon ginger, grated

- **Instructions:**

1. Heat olive oil in a large pan over medium heat. Add the garlic and ginger, sautéing until fragrant.

2. Add the chicken slices and cook until browned and cooked through.

3. Add the broccoli florets and soy sauce, cooking until the broccoli is tender.

4. Serve the stir-fry over the cooked brown rice.

- **Benefits:**

- This dish is high in protein and fiber, making it a balanced and wholesome dinner option.

6. Butternut Squash and Sage Risotto

- **Ingredients:**
    - 1 cup Arborio rice
    - 1 cup butternut squash, diced
    - 4 cups low-sodium vegetable broth, warmed
    - 1/4 cup lactose-free parmesan cheese, grated
    - 2 tablespoons olive oil
    - 1 small onion, finely chopped
    - 1 tablespoon fresh sage, chopped
    - Salt and pepper to taste
- **Instructions:**

1. In a large pan, heat the olive oil over medium heat and sauté the onion until softened.

2. Add the butternut squash and cook until slightly softened.

3. Add the Arborio rice and stir for 2-3 minutes until the rice is lightly toasted.

4. Gradually add the warm vegetable broth, one ladleful at a time, stirring constantly until the liquid is absorbed before adding more.

5. Continue cooking and stirring until the rice is creamy and tender, about 20-25 minutes in total.

6. Stir in the grated parmesan cheese and fresh sage. Season with salt and pepper.

7. Serve warm for a comforting and flavorful meal.

- **Benefits:**
    - This risotto is rich in vitamins A and C, making it a nourishing and antioxidant-packed dinner.

7. Garlic Parmesan Pasta

- **Ingredients:**
    - 8 oz penne pasta (softened)
    - 1/2 cup lactose-free parmesan cheese, grated
    - 4 cloves garlic, minced
    - 1/4 cup olive oil
    - 1/4 cup fresh parsley, chopped
    - Salt and pepper to taste
- **Instructions:**

1. Cook the penne pasta according to package instructions. Drain and set aside.

2. In a large pan, heat the olive oil over medium heat and sauté the garlic until golden.

3. Toss the cooked pasta in the garlic and olive oil, coating it well.

4. Stir in the grated parmesan cheese and season with salt and pepper.

5. Garnish with fresh parsley and serve warm.

- **Benefits:**
  - This pasta dish is simple, yet flavorful, providing a good source of calcium and healthy fats.

8. Vegetable Fried Rice

- **Ingredients:**
  - 2 cups cooked brown rice
  - 1/2 cup carrots, diced
  - 1/2 cup peas
  - 1/2 cup bell peppers, diced
  - 2 tablespoons soy sauce (low sodium)
  - 1 tablespoon olive oil
  - 2 eggs, lightly beaten

- 2 cloves garlic, minced

- **Instructions:**

1. Heat the olive oil in a large pan over medium heat. Add the garlic and sauté until fragrant.

2. Add the carrots, peas, and bell peppers, cooking until tender.

3. Push the vegetables to the side of the pan and pour in the beaten eggs, scrambling them until fully cooked.

4. Stir in the cooked rice and soy sauce, mixing everything together.

5. Serve warm for a quick and nutritious meal.

- **Benefits:**
  - This fried rice is packed with vegetables and protein, making it a balanced and flavorful dinner option.

9. Pasta Primavera

- **Ingredients:**
  - 8 oz penne pasta (softened)
  - 1 cup zucchini, sliced
  - 1 cup cherry tomatoes, halved
  - 1/2 cup bell peppers, sliced
  - 1/2 cup peas

- 1/4 cup olive oil
- 1/4 cup lactose-free parmesan cheese, grated
- 2 cloves garlic, minced
- Salt and pepper to taste

- **Instructions:**

1. Cook the penne pasta according to package instructions. Drain and set aside.

2. In a large pan, heat the olive oil over medium heat and sauté the garlic until fragrant.

3. Add the zucchini, cherry tomatoes, bell peppers, and peas, cooking until the vegetables are tender.

4. Toss the cooked pasta in the vegetables and olive oil.

5. Stir in the grated parmesan cheese and season with salt and pepper.

6. Serve warm with a sprinkle of extra parmesan cheese.

- **Benefits:**
  - This dish is rich in vitamins and minerals, offering a colorful and nutrient-dense meal.

10. Baked Ziti with Ground Turkey

- **Ingredients:**

- 8 oz ziti pasta (softened)
- 1/2 pound ground turkey
- 1 cup marinara sauce (low sodium)
- 1/2 cup lactose-free mozzarella cheese, shredded
- 1/4 cup lactose-free ricotta cheese
- 1 tablespoon olive oil
- 1 small onion, chopped
- 2 cloves garlic, minced
- Salt and pepper to taste

- **Instructions:**

1. Preheat the oven to 375°F (190°C).

2. Cook the ziti pasta according to package instructions. Drain and set aside.

3. In a large pan, heat the olive oil over medium heat. Add the onion and garlic, sautéing until softened.

4. Add the ground turkey and cook until browned.

5. Stir in the marinara sauce and season with salt and pepper.

6. In a large baking dish, layer the cooked ziti pasta, turkey marinara sauce, ricotta cheese, and shredded mozzarella.

7. Bake for 20-25 minutes, or until the cheese is melted and bubbly.

8. Serve hot for a comforting and hearty meal.

- **Benefits:**
    - This baked ziti is high in protein and calcium, providing a satisfying and filling dinner option.

Tender Meat and Fish Entrées

This section focuses on tender, easy-to-digest meat and fish entrées that are perfect for dinner during your ileostomy recovery. These recipes are designed to be both gentle on your digestive system and rich in essential nutrients to support your healing process.

1. Herb-Roasted Chicken Breast

- **Ingredients:**
    - 2 chicken breasts
    - 2 tablespoons olive oil
    - 1 tablespoon fresh rosemary, chopped
    - 1 tablespoon fresh thyme, chopped
    - 2 cloves garlic, minced

- Salt and pepper to taste

- **Instructions:**

1. Preheat the oven to 375°F (190°C).

2. In a small bowl, mix together the olive oil, rosemary, thyme, garlic, salt, and pepper.

3. Rub the mixture evenly over the chicken breasts.

4. Place the chicken on a baking sheet and roast for 25-30 minutes, or until the chicken is cooked through and tender.

5. Serve warm with a side of soft vegetables or mashed potatoes.

- **Benefits:**
  - This dish provides lean protein and is flavored with fresh herbs, making it a simple and nutritious option for dinner.

2. Lemon Dill Baked Salmon

- **Ingredients:**
  - 2 salmon fillets
  - 2 tablespoons olive oil
  - 2 tablespoons fresh dill, chopped
  - 1 lemon, sliced
  - Salt and pepper to taste

- **Instructions:**

1. Preheat the oven to 375°F (190°C).

2. Place the salmon fillets on a baking sheet lined with parchment paper.

3. Drizzle the olive oil over the salmon and sprinkle with dill, salt, and pepper.

4. Place the lemon slices on top of the salmon.

5. Bake for 15-20 minutes, or until the salmon is cooked through and flakes easily with a fork.

6. Serve warm with a side of soft rice or steamed vegetables.

- **Benefits:**
  - Salmon is rich in omega-3 fatty acids, which are anti-inflammatory and support overall health during recovery.

3. Slow-Cooked Beef Brisket

- **Ingredients:**
  - 1 pound beef brisket
  - 1 cup low-sodium beef broth
  - 1 onion, sliced
  - 2 cloves garlic, minced
  - 1 tablespoon olive oil

- o 1 teaspoon thyme
- o Salt and pepper to taste

- **Instructions:**

1. Heat the olive oil in a large pan over medium heat and sear the brisket on all sides until browned.

2. Transfer the brisket to a slow cooker.

3. Add the onion, garlic, beef broth, thyme, salt, and pepper to the slow cooker.

4. Cook on low for 6-8 hours, or until the brisket is tender and falls apart easily.

5. Serve warm with a side of mashed potatoes or soft-cooked vegetables.

- **Benefits:**
  - o Slow-cooked brisket is incredibly tender and easy to digest, making it a hearty and comforting meal option.

4. Poached Cod with Lemon Butter Sauce

- **Ingredients:**
  - o 2 cod fillets
  - o 2 cups low-sodium vegetable broth
  - o 1 lemon, juiced
  - o 2 tablespoons unsalted butter

- o   1 tablespoon fresh parsley, chopped
- o   Salt and pepper to taste
- **Instructions:**

1. In a large skillet, bring the vegetable broth to a simmer over medium heat.

2. Add the cod fillets to the skillet and poach for 5-7 minutes, or until the fish is opaque and flakes easily with a fork.

3. In a small saucepan, melt the butter and stir in the lemon juice and parsley.

4. Carefully remove the cod from the skillet and drizzle with the lemon butter sauce.

5. Serve warm with a side of soft rice or steamed vegetables.

- **Benefits:**
  - o   Poached cod is light and easy to digest, and the lemon butter sauce adds a refreshing flavor without being too heavy.

5. Turkey Meatballs in Tomato Sauce

- **Ingredients:**
  - o   1/2 pound ground turkey
  - o   1/4 cup breadcrumbs (gluten-free if needed)

- 1 egg, lightly beaten
- 2 tablespoons fresh parsley, chopped
- 2 cups low-sodium tomato sauce
- 1 tablespoon olive oil
- Salt and pepper to taste

- **Instructions:**

1. Preheat the oven to 375°F (190°C).

2. In a large bowl, combine the ground turkey, breadcrumbs, egg, parsley, salt, and pepper. Mix well.

3. Shape the mixture into small meatballs and place them on a baking sheet.

4. Bake for 15-20 minutes, or until the meatballs are cooked through.

5. In a large pan, heat the tomato sauce over medium heat.

6. Add the cooked meatballs to the sauce and simmer for 10 minutes.

7. Serve warm over soft pasta or rice.

- **Benefits:**
  - These turkey meatballs are high in protein and easy to digest, making them a versatile and satisfying dinner option.

6. Chicken Piccata

- **Ingredients:**
    - 2 chicken breasts, thinly sliced
    - 1/4 cup all-purpose flour (gluten-free if needed)
    - 1/4 cup low-sodium chicken broth
    - 1/4 cup lemon juice
    - 2 tablespoons capers, rinsed
    - 2 tablespoons olive oil
    - Salt and pepper to taste
- **Instructions:**

1. Lightly coat the chicken breasts in flour, shaking off any excess.

2. In a large pan, heat the olive oil over medium heat and cook the chicken until golden brown on both sides.

3. Add the chicken broth, lemon juice, and capers to the pan, bringing the mixture to a simmer.

4. Cook for 5-7 minutes, or until the sauce has thickened slightly and the chicken is cooked through.

5. Serve warm with a side of soft vegetables or rice.

- **Benefits:**

- Chicken piccata is light, flavorful, and easy to digest, providing a balanced meal that's perfect for dinner.

7. Baked Tilapia with Garlic and Herbs

- **Ingredients:**
    - 2 tilapia fillets
    - 2 tablespoons olive oil
    - 2 cloves garlic, minced
    - 1 tablespoon fresh parsley, chopped
    - 1 tablespoon fresh thyme, chopped
    - Salt and pepper to taste
- **Instructions:**

1. Preheat the oven to 375°F (190°C).
2. Place the tilapia fillets on a baking sheet lined with parchment paper.
3. Drizzle the olive oil over the fillets and sprinkle with garlic, parsley, thyme, salt, and pepper.
4. Bake for 15-20 minutes, or until the tilapia is cooked through and flakes easily with a fork.
5. Serve warm with a side of soft rice or steamed vegetables.

- **Benefits:**

- Tilapia is a mild-flavored fish that is easy to digest, making it a great choice for a light and healthy dinner.

8. Pork Tenderloin with Apple Sauce

- **Ingredients:**
    - 1 pound pork tenderloin
    - 2 apples, peeled and sliced
    - 1/2 cup unsweetened applesauce
    - 1 tablespoon olive oil
    - 1 tablespoon fresh rosemary, chopped
    - Salt and pepper to taste
- **Instructions:**

1. Preheat the oven to 375°F (190°C).
2. Season the pork tenderloin with rosemary, salt, and pepper.
3. In a large oven-safe pan, heat the olive oil over medium heat and sear the pork tenderloin on all sides until browned.
4. Add the sliced apples to the pan and transfer to the oven.
5. Roast for 20-25 minutes, or until the pork is cooked through.

6. Slice the pork and serve with the applesauce and roasted apples.

- **Benefits:**
    - Pork tenderloin is a lean protein source, and the apples provide a natural sweetness that complements the meat, making it easy to digest.

9. Lemon Herb Chicken Thighs

- **Ingredients:**
    - 4 chicken thighs, skinless
    - 1/4 cup olive oil
    - 1/4 cup lemon juice
    - 1 tablespoon fresh thyme, chopped
    - 1 tablespoon fresh rosemary, chopped
    - 2 cloves garlic, minced
    - Salt and pepper to taste
- **Instructions:**

1. In a large bowl, combine the olive oil, lemon juice, thyme, rosemary, garlic, salt, and pepper.

2. Add the chicken thighs and marinate for at least 30 minutes.

3. Preheat the oven to 375°F (190°C).

4. Place the chicken thighs on a baking sheet and bake for 30-35 minutes, or until the chicken is cooked through and tender.

5. Serve warm with a side of soft vegetables or rice.

- **Benefits:**
    - Chicken thighs are flavorful and juicy, and when paired with fresh herbs and lemon, they make a delicious and easy-to-digest meal.

10. Braised Lamb Shanks

- **Ingredients:**
    - 2 lamb shanks
    - 2 cups low-sodium beef broth
    - 1 onion, chopped
    - 2 cloves garlic, minced
    - 1 tablespoon olive oil
    - 1 teaspoon fresh rosemary, chopped
    - Salt and pepper to taste
- **Instructions:**

1. Preheat the oven to 325°F (160°C).

2.   Heat the olive oil in a large oven-safe pan over medium heat. Sear the lamb shanks on all sides until browned.

3.   Add the onion, garlic, beef broth, rosemary, salt, and pepper to the pan.

4.   Cover the pan and transfer to the oven.

5.   Braise for 2-3 hours, or until the lamb is tender and falls off the bone.

6.   Serve warm with a side of mashed potatoes or soft-cooked vegetables.

- **Benefits:**
  - Braised lamb shanks are tender and rich in flavor, providing a hearty and satisfying meal that's easy to digest.

<u>Veggie-Centric Options for Plant-Based Delights</u>

This section offers a variety of plant-based dinner recipes that are both nourishing and easy on your digestive system. These veggie-centric dishes are designed to provide essential nutrients while being gentle on your ileostomy recovery.

1. Stuffed Bell Peppers

- **Ingredients:**
    - 4 large bell peppers, tops cut off and seeds removed
    - 1 cup cooked quinoa
    - 1 cup black beans, rinsed and drained
    - 1 cup corn kernels
    - 1/2 cup lactose-free shredded cheese
    - 1 small onion, chopped
    - 1 clove garlic, minced
    - 1 tablespoon olive oil
    - Salt and pepper to taste
- **Instructions:**

1. Preheat the oven to 375°F (190°C).

2. In a large pan, heat the olive oil over medium heat. Sauté the onion and garlic until softened.

3. Stir in the cooked quinoa, black beans, corn, salt, and pepper.

4. Stuff the bell peppers with the quinoa mixture and place them in a baking dish.

5. Top each stuffed pepper with shredded cheese.

6. Bake for 25-30 minutes, or until the peppers are tender and the cheese is melted.

7. Serve warm as a complete meal.

- **Benefits:**
    - This dish is high in fiber, protein, and vitamins, offering a balanced plant-based meal that's filling and easy to digest.

2. Zucchini Noodles with Pesto

- **Ingredients:**
    - 4 medium zucchinis, spiralized into noodles
    - 1/4 cup fresh basil leaves
    - 1/4 cup fresh parsley
    - 1/4 cup pine nuts
    - 2 cloves garlic, minced
    - 1/4 cup olive oil
    - Salt and pepper to taste
- **Instructions:**

1. In a food processor, combine basil, parsley, pine nuts, garlic, and olive oil. Blend until smooth. Season with salt and pepper.

2. In a large pan, heat a small amount of olive oil over medium heat. Add the zucchini noodles and sauté for 2-3 minutes until slightly softened.

3. Remove from heat and toss the zucchini noodles with the pesto sauce.

4. Serve warm, garnished with extra pine nuts or a sprinkle of lactose-free parmesan cheese.

- **Benefits:**
    - Zucchini noodles are low in carbs and easy to digest, while the pesto adds a burst of flavor and healthy fats.

3. Butternut Squash Risotto

- **Ingredients:**
    - 1 cup arborio rice
    - 2 cups butternut squash, peeled and cubed
    - 4 cups low-sodium vegetable broth
    - 1/2 cup lactose-free parmesan cheese, grated
    - 1 small onion, chopped
    - 2 cloves garlic, minced
    - 2 tablespoons olive oil
    - Salt and pepper to taste
- **Instructions:**

1. In a large pot, heat the olive oil over medium heat. Sauté the onion and garlic until softened.

2. Add the arborio rice and stir to coat with the oil.

3. Slowly add the vegetable broth, one cup at a time, stirring frequently until absorbed.

4. Meanwhile, steam the butternut squash until tender, then mash it lightly with a fork.

5. Stir the mashed squash into the risotto and continue cooking until the rice is tender and creamy.

6. Stir in the grated parmesan cheese and season with salt and pepper.

7. Serve warm as a comforting and nutritious meal.

- **Benefits:**
    - This risotto is creamy and rich in flavor, with the butternut squash providing a good source of vitamins A and C.

4. Cauliflower and Sweet Potato Curry

- **Ingredients:**
    - 1 small cauliflower, cut into florets
    - 2 medium sweet potatoes, peeled and cubed
    - 1 can (14 oz) coconut milk
    - 1 cup low-sodium vegetable broth

- 1 small onion, chopped
- 2 cloves garlic, minced
- 1 tablespoon curry powder
- 1 tablespoon olive oil
- Salt and pepper to taste

- **Instructions:**

1. In a large pot, heat the olive oil over medium heat. Sauté the onion and garlic until softened.

2. Add the curry powder and cook for 1 minute, stirring constantly.

3. Add the cauliflower and sweet potatoes, stirring to coat with the spices.

4. Pour in the coconut milk and vegetable broth, bringing the mixture to a simmer.

5. Cover and cook for 20-25 minutes, or until the vegetables are tender.

6. Season with salt and pepper to taste and serve warm over soft rice.

- **Benefits:**
  - This curry is packed with anti-inflammatory properties from the turmeric and other spices, and the vegetables provide a hearty and satisfying meal.

5. Eggplant Parmesan (Baked)

- **Ingredients:**
    - 2 medium eggplants, sliced into rounds
    - 1 cup marinara sauce (low sodium)
    - 1/2 cup lactose-free mozzarella cheese, shredded
    - 1/4 cup lactose-free parmesan cheese, grated
    - 1/2 cup breadcrumbs (gluten-free if needed)
    - 2 tablespoons olive oil
    - Salt and pepper to taste
- **Instructions:**

1. Preheat the oven to 375°F (190°C).
2. Lightly brush the eggplant slices with olive oil and season with salt and pepper.
3. In a shallow dish, coat the eggplant slices in breadcrumbs.
4. Place the eggplant slices on a baking sheet and bake for 15-20 minutes, or until golden brown.
5. In a baking dish, layer the baked eggplant slices with marinara sauce and shredded mozzarella.
6. Sprinkle the top with grated parmesan cheese.

7. Bake for an additional 15-20 minutes, or until the cheese is melted and bubbly.

8. Serve warm with a side of soft pasta.

- **Benefits:**
    - This baked eggplant parmesan is a healthier, lower-fat alternative to the traditional fried version, offering a satisfying, plant-based entrée.

6. Spinach and Ricotta Stuffed Shells

- **Ingredients:**
    - 12 jumbo pasta shells (gluten-free if needed)
    - 1 cup spinach, steamed and chopped
    - 1/2 cup lactose-free ricotta cheese
    - 1/2 cup lactose-free mozzarella cheese, shredded
    - 1 cup marinara sauce (low sodium)
    - 1 tablespoon olive oil
    - Salt and pepper to taste
- **Instructions:**

1. Preheat the oven to 375°F (190°C).

2. Cook the pasta shells according to package instructions. Drain and set aside.

3. In a bowl, mix together the chopped spinach, ricotta cheese, salt, and pepper.

4. Stuff each pasta shell with the spinach and ricotta mixture.

5. In a baking dish, spread a thin layer of marinara sauce.

6. Arrange the stuffed shells in the dish and top with the remaining marinara sauce and shredded mozzarella.

7. Bake for 20-25 minutes, or until the cheese is melted and the dish is heated through.

8. Serve warm as a comforting and filling meal.

- **Benefits:**
  - This dish is rich in calcium and protein, making it a nourishing option that's easy on the stomach.

7. Mushroom and Barley Stew

- **Ingredients:**
  - 1 cup pearl barley
  - 2 cups mushrooms, sliced
  - 1 small onion, chopped
  - 2 cloves garlic, minced
  - 4 cups low-sodium vegetable broth

- 1 tablespoon olive oil
- 1 teaspoon thyme
- Salt and pepper to taste

- **Instructions:**

1. In a large pot, heat the olive oil over medium heat. Sauté the onion, garlic, and mushrooms until softened.

2. Add the barley and stir to coat with the oil.

3. Pour in the vegetable broth and add thyme, salt, and pepper.

4. Bring the mixture to a boil, then reduce heat and simmer for 30-40 minutes, or until the barley is tender.

5. Serve warm as a hearty and filling stew.

- **Benefits:**
  - This stew is rich in fiber and nutrients, making it a hearty, plant-based meal that supports digestive health.

8. Sweet Potato and Black Bean Enchiladas

- **Ingredients:**
  - 4 large tortillas (gluten-free if needed)
  - 2 medium sweet potatoes, peeled and cubed
  - 1 cup black beans, rinsed and drained

- 1 cup enchilada sauce (low sodium)
- 1/2 cup lactose-free shredded cheese
- 1 small onion, chopped
- 1 tablespoon olive oil
- Salt and pepper to taste

- **Instructions:**

1. Preheat the oven to 375°F (190°C).
2. In a large pan, heat the olive oil over medium heat. Sauté the onion until softened.
3. Add the sweet potatoes and cook until tender, then stir in the black beans, salt, and pepper.
4. Place a portion of the sweet potato mixture in the center of each tortilla and roll up.
5. Arrange the tortillas in a baking dish and pour the enchilada sauce over the top.
6. Sprinkle with shredded cheese.
7. Bake for 20-25 minutes, or until the cheese is melted and the enchiladas are heated through.
8. Serve warm with a side of steamed vegetables.

- **Benefits:**

- These enchiladas are a flavorful and filling dish that's packed with protein and fiber, supporting overall digestive health.

9. Carrot and Ginger Soup

- **Ingredients:**
  - 4 large carrots, peeled and chopped
  - 1 small onion, chopped
  - 2 cloves garlic, minced
  - 4 cups low-sodium vegetable broth
  - 1 tablespoon fresh ginger, grated
  - 1 tablespoon olive oil
  - Salt and pepper to taste
- **Instructions:**

1. In a large pot, heat the olive oil over medium heat. Sauté the onion, garlic, and ginger until softened.

2. Add the carrots and vegetable broth, bringing the mixture to a boil.

3. Reduce heat and simmer for 20-25 minutes, or until the carrots are tender.

4. Use an immersion blender to puree the soup until smooth.

5. Season with salt and pepper and serve warm.

- **Benefits:**
  - This soup is rich in beta-carotene and anti-inflammatory properties, making it a soothing and nutrient-dense option.

10. **Roasted Vegetable and Quinoa Bowl**

- **Ingredients:**
  - 1 cup quinoa, cooked
  - 1 zucchini, sliced
  - 1 bell pepper, sliced
  - 1 cup cherry tomatoes, halved
  - 1 small onion, sliced
  - 2 tablespoons olive oil
  - 1 tablespoon balsamic vinegar
  - Salt and pepper to taste
- **Instructions:**

1. Preheat the oven to 400°F (200°C).

2. In a large bowl, toss the zucchini, bell pepper, cherry tomatoes, and onion with olive oil, balsamic vinegar, salt, and pepper.

3. Spread the vegetables on a baking sheet and roast for 20-25 minutes, or until tender and slightly caramelized.

4. Serve the roasted vegetables over cooked quinoa.
- **Benefits:**
  - This bowl is a balanced and filling meal, packed with vitamins, minerals, and plant-based protein.

Chapter 7: Snacks and Sides to Support Your Diet

Crunchy and Chewy Snack Ideas

These snack ideas are perfect for when you need something light between meals. They offer a balance of textures and flavors while being gentle on your digestive system.

1. Baked Apple Chips

- **Ingredients:**
    - 2 apples, thinly sliced
    - 1 teaspoon cinnamon
    - 1 tablespoon honey (optional)
- **Instructions:**

1. Preheat the oven to 225°F (110°C).

2. Arrange the apple slices on a parchment-lined baking sheet.

3. Sprinkle with cinnamon and drizzle with honey, if desired.

4. Bake for 1.5-2 hours, flipping halfway through, until the apples are crisp.

5. Let cool and enjoy as a crunchy snack.

- **Benefits:**
    - Apples are high in fiber and antioxidants, making these chips a healthy, satisfying snack.

2. Crispy Chickpeas

- **Ingredients:**
    - 1 can (15 oz) chickpeas, drained and rinsed
    - 1 tablespoon olive oil
    - 1/2 teaspoon paprika
    - 1/2 teaspoon garlic powder
    - Salt to taste
- **Instructions:**

1. Preheat the oven to 400°F (200°C).
2. Pat the chickpeas dry with a paper towel and spread them on a baking sheet.
3. Drizzle with olive oil and sprinkle with paprika, garlic powder, and salt.
4. Roast for 25-30 minutes, shaking the pan occasionally, until the chickpeas are crispy.
5. Let cool and enjoy as a crunchy, protein-packed snack.

- **Benefits:**

- Chickpeas are rich in protein and fiber, providing a crunchy snack that supports digestive health.

3. Soft Banana Oat Bars

- **Ingredients:**
    - 2 ripe bananas, mashed
    - 1 cup rolled oats
    - 1/4 cup almond butter
    - 1/4 cup honey
    - 1/4 cup raisins (optional)
- **Instructions:**

1. Preheat the oven to 350°F (175°C).
2. In a bowl, combine the mashed bananas, oats, almond butter, honey, and raisins.
3. Press the mixture into a greased 8x8-inch baking dish.
4. Bake for 15-20 minutes, or until the bars are set and lightly browned.
5. Let cool before cutting into squares.

- **Benefits:**
    - These bars are chewy and naturally sweet, offering a quick and nutritious snack.

4. Yogurt-Dipped Strawberries

- **Ingredients:**
    - 1 cup strawberries, washed and hulled
    - 1/2 cup lactose-free Greek yogurt
    - 1 tablespoon honey (optional)
- **Instructions:**

1. Dip each strawberry into the yogurt, coating it evenly.
2. Place the dipped strawberries on a parchment-lined tray.
3. Freeze for at least 1 hour before serving.

- **Benefits:**
    - This snack combines the sweetness of strawberries with the creaminess of yogurt, offering a refreshing and light treat.

5. Soft Granola Bites

- **Ingredients:**
    - 1 cup rolled oats
    - 1/4 cup almond butter
    - 1/4 cup honey
    - 1/4 cup dried cranberries

- 1/4 cup sunflower seeds

- **Instructions:**

1. In a large bowl, mix all the ingredients until well combined.

2. Roll the mixture into small balls and place them on a parchment-lined tray.

3. Refrigerate for at least 30 minutes before serving.

- **Benefits:**
    - These granola bites are packed with energy-boosting ingredients, perfect for a quick, nutritious snack.

Satisfying Side Dishes for Every Meal

These side dishes are designed to complement your main meals, providing additional nutrients and flavors while being easy on your digestive system.

1. Mashed Sweet Potatoes

- **Ingredients:**
    - 2 large sweet potatoes, peeled and cubed
    - 1/4 cup lactose-free milk
    - 2 tablespoons butter
    - Salt and pepper to taste

- **Instructions:**

1. Boil the sweet potatoes in a pot of water until tender, about 15-20 minutes.

2. Drain and mash the sweet potatoes with the milk, butter, salt, and pepper.

3. Serve warm as a comforting and nutritious side dish.

- **Benefits:**
  - Sweet potatoes are high in vitamins A and C, offering a smooth and satisfying side.

2. Steamed Green Beans with Olive Oil

- **Ingredients:**
  - 2 cups fresh green beans, trimmed
  - 1 tablespoon olive oil
  - 1 teaspoon lemon juice
  - Salt and pepper to taste

- **Instructions:**

1. Steam the green beans until tender but still crisp, about 5-7 minutes.

2. Drizzle with olive oil and lemon juice, then season with salt and pepper.

3. Serve warm or at room temperature.

- **Benefits:**
    - Green beans are rich in fiber and vitamins, making them a light and nutritious side dish.

3. Creamy Polenta

- **Ingredients:**
    - 1 cup cornmeal
    - 4 cups water
    - 1/4 cup lactose-free parmesan cheese, grated
    - 2 tablespoons butter
    - Salt to taste
- **Instructions:**

1. Bring the water to a boil in a large pot.
2. Gradually whisk in the cornmeal, reducing the heat to low.
3. Cook, stirring frequently, until the polenta is thick and creamy, about 20 minutes.
4. Stir in the parmesan cheese, butter, and salt.
5. Serve warm as a smooth and comforting side dish.

- **Benefits:**

- Polenta is a gentle and easy-to-digest side, providing a warm and filling addition to any meal.

Homemade Dips and Spreads

These dips and spreads are perfect for pairing with soft vegetables, crackers, or bread, offering a flavorful addition to your snacks and meals.

1. Classic Hummus

- **Ingredients:**
    - 1 can (15 oz) chickpeas, drained and rinsed
    - 1/4 cup tahini
    - 2 cloves garlic, minced
    - 2 tablespoons lemon juice
    - 2 tablespoons olive oil
    - Salt to taste
- **Instructions:**

1. In a food processor, combine the chickpeas, tahini, garlic, lemon juice, and olive oil.

2. Blend until smooth, adding a little water if needed to reach the desired consistency.

3. Season with salt and serve with soft pita bread or vegetable sticks.

- **Benefits:**
    - Hummus is rich in protein and healthy fats, making it a nutritious and versatile spread.

2. Avocado and Yogurt Dip

- **Ingredients:**
    - 2 ripe avocados, pitted and peeled
    - 1/2 cup lactose-free Greek yogurt
    - 1 tablespoon lime juice
    - Salt and pepper to taste
- **Instructions:**

1. Mash the avocados in a bowl.

2. Stir in the yogurt, lime juice, salt, and pepper until well combined.

3. Serve as a creamy dip with soft crackers or bread.

- **Benefits:**
    - This dip is packed with healthy fats and probiotics, offering a creamy and nutritious option.

Nutrient-Rich Trail Mixes and Bars

These homemade trail mixes and bars provide a quick and easy way to get a nutrient boost, perfect for when you're on the go.

1. Nut and Seed Trail Mix

- **Ingredients:**
    - 1/2 cup almonds
    - 1/2 cup cashews
    - 1/4 cup sunflower seeds
    - 1/4 cup pumpkin seeds
    - 1/4 cup dried cranberries
- **Instructions:**

1. Mix all the ingredients in a large bowl.
2. Store in an airtight container for a convenient, on-the-go snack.

- **Benefits:**
    - This trail mix is rich in healthy fats, protein, and fiber, providing sustained energy.

2. Peanut Butter Protein Bars

- **Ingredients:**
    - 1 cup rolled oats

- 1/2 cup peanut butter
- 1/4 cup honey
- 1/4 cup protein powder
- 1/4 cup dark chocolate chips (optional)

- **Instructions:**

1. In a bowl, mix together the oats, peanut butter, honey, protein powder, and chocolate chips.

2. Press the mixture into a greased 8x8-inch baking dish.

3. Refrigerate for at least 30 minutes before cutting into bars.

- **Benefits:**
  - These bars are packed with protein and healthy fats, making them a filling and nutritious snack.

Chapter 8: Desserts for Sweet Indulgences

Soft and Decadent Puddings

These pudding recipes are creamy, smooth, and gentle on the digestive system, offering a perfect way to satisfy your sweet tooth without causing discomfort.

1. Classic Vanilla Pudding

- **Ingredients:**
    - 2 cups lactose-free milk
    - 1/2 cup sugar
    - 3 tablespoons cornstarch
    - 1/4 teaspoon salt
    - 1 teaspoon vanilla extract
- **Instructions:**

1. In a medium saucepan, whisk together the sugar, cornstarch, and salt.

2. Gradually whisk in the milk until smooth.

3. Cook over medium heat, stirring constantly, until the mixture thickens and comes to a gentle boil.

4. Remove from heat and stir in the vanilla extract.

5. Pour into serving dishes and let cool before refrigerating for at least 2 hours.

- **Benefits:**
    - This pudding is light and easy to digest, making it a comforting dessert option that's still satisfying.

2. Chocolate Avocado Pudding

- **Ingredients:**
    - 2 ripe avocados, peeled and pitted
    - 1/4 cup cocoa powder
    - 1/4 cup honey or maple syrup
    - 1/4 cup lactose-free milk
    - 1 teaspoon vanilla extract
- **Instructions:**

1. In a blender, combine the avocados, cocoa powder, honey, milk, and vanilla extract.

2. Blend until smooth and creamy.

3. Spoon the pudding into serving dishes and refrigerate for at least 1 hour before serving.

- **Benefits:**

- Rich in healthy fats and antioxidants, this pudding is a guilt-free indulgence that supports overall health.

3. Banana Chia Pudding

- **Ingredients:**
  - 2 ripe bananas, mashed
  - 1/4 cup chia seeds
  - 1 1/2 cups lactose-free milk
  - 1 teaspoon vanilla extract
  - 1 tablespoon honey (optional)
- **Instructions:**

1. In a bowl, mix together the mashed bananas, chia seeds, milk, vanilla extract, and honey.

2. Stir well and let the mixture sit for 5 minutes.

3. Stir again to prevent the chia seeds from clumping, then cover and refrigerate for at least 4 hours or overnight.

4. Serve chilled, optionally topped with sliced bananas or a sprinkle of cinnamon.

- **Benefits:**

- Chia seeds are a great source of fiber and omega-3 fatty acids, making this pudding both nutritious and satisfying.

Fruity Sorbets and Gelatin Treats

These light and refreshing desserts are made with natural fruit flavors, providing a cool and sweet end to any meal.

1. Strawberry Lemon Sorbet

- **Ingredients:**
    - 2 cups fresh strawberries, hulled
    - 1/2 cup sugar
    - 1/2 cup water
    - 2 tablespoons lemon juice
- **Instructions:**

1. In a blender, puree the strawberries until smooth.

2. In a small saucepan, combine the sugar and water, heating until the sugar dissolves to make a simple syrup.

3. Stir the lemon juice into the strawberry puree, then add the simple syrup.

4. Pour the mixture into a shallow dish and freeze, stirring every 30 minutes until fully frozen.

5. Scoop into bowls and serve.

- **Benefits:**
    - This sorbet is light, refreshing, and made with real fruit, making it a healthy, low-calorie dessert.

2. Orange Gelatin Delight

- **Ingredients:**
    - 2 cups freshly squeezed orange juice
    - 1 tablespoon gelatin powder
    - 2 tablespoons honey or agave syrup
- **Instructions:**

1. In a small saucepan, heat 1 cup of the orange juice until warm but not boiling.

2. Sprinkle the gelatin over the juice and stir until fully dissolved.

3. Remove from heat and stir in the remaining orange juice and honey.

4. Pour the mixture into serving dishes and refrigerate until set, about 4 hours.

5. Serve chilled.

- **Benefits:**

- This gelatin treat is hydrating and packed with vitamin C, making it a simple and nourishing dessert.

Baked Goods Made Easy on the Digestive System

These baked treats are designed to be gentle on your system, with ingredients that are easy to digest while still offering the comforting flavors you crave.

1. Oatmeal Cookies

- **Ingredients:**
    - 1 cup rolled oats
    - 1/2 cup almond flour
    - 1/4 cup honey or maple syrup
    - 1/4 cup coconut oil, melted
    - 1/2 teaspoon vanilla extract
    - 1/4 teaspoon baking soda
    - 1/4 cup raisins (optional)
- **Instructions:**

1. Preheat the oven to 350°F (175°C).

2. In a large bowl, mix together all ingredients until well combined.

3. Drop spoonfuls of the dough onto a parchment-lined baking sheet.

4. Bake for 10-12 minutes, or until the edges are lightly golden.

5. Let cool before serving.

- **Benefits:**
    - These cookies are made with whole grains and natural sweeteners, providing a treat that's easy on your stomach and satisfying.

2. Pumpkin Muffins

- **Ingredients:**
    - 1 cup pumpkin puree
    - 1/2 cup almond flour
    - 1/4 cup coconut sugar
    - 2 eggs
    - 1 teaspoon cinnamon
    - 1/2 teaspoon baking powder
    - 1/4 teaspoon baking soda
- **Instructions:**

1. Preheat the oven to 350°F (175°C).

2. In a bowl, mix together the pumpkin puree, almond flour, coconut sugar, eggs, cinnamon, baking powder, and baking soda until well combined.

3. Divide the batter into a greased muffin tin.

4. Bake for 18-20 minutes, or until a toothpick inserted into the center comes out clean.

5. Let cool before serving.

- **Benefits:**
    - These muffins are rich in fiber and beta-carotene, offering a sweet and nutritious snack or dessert.

Guilt-Free Dessert Alternatives

These dessert alternatives are designed to satisfy your sweet cravings without the extra calories, sugar, or fat, making them perfect for maintaining a balanced diet.

1. Greek Yogurt with Honey and Berries

- **Ingredients:**
    - 1 cup lactose-free Greek yogurt
    - 1 tablespoon honey
    - 1/2 cup mixed berries (such as strawberries, blueberries, and raspberries)

- **Instructions:**
1. Spoon the Greek yogurt into a bowl.
2. Drizzle with honey and top with mixed berries.
3. Serve immediately.
- **Benefits:**
    - This dessert is packed with protein, probiotics, and antioxidants, making it both delicious and beneficial for your digestive health.

2. Frozen Banana Bites

- **Ingredients:**
    - 2 ripe bananas
    - 1/4 cup dark chocolate, melted
    - 1 tablespoon chopped nuts or coconut flakes (optional)
- **Instructions:**
1. Slice the bananas into bite-sized pieces.
2. Dip each piece into the melted dark chocolate and place on a parchment-lined tray.
3. Sprinkle with chopped nuts or coconut flakes, if desired.
4. Freeze for at least 1 hour before serving.

- **Benefits:**
    - These banana bites are a simple, naturally sweet treat that's rich in potassium and fiber, supporting overall health.

Conclusion

As you reach the end of "The Ileostomy Diet Cookbook for newly diagnosed," we hope you find yourself better equipped to embark on your journey to health and wellness with your ileostomy. The recipes and meal plans provided are designed not only to meet your dietary needs but also to make your recovery process smoother and more enjoyable.

Navigating life with an ileostomy can be a significant adjustment, but with the right dietary approach, you can thrive. By focusing on gentle, nourishing foods and understanding the role of diet in your recovery, you can enhance your comfort, support your digestive system, and enjoy a diverse range of delicious meals. Remember, each meal you prepare is a step towards a healthier, more vibrant you.

Your journey doesn't end with these recipes. Embrace the flexibility and creativity that cooking offers, adapting recipes to fit your personal tastes and dietary needs. Continue to explore and learn about foods that work best for your body, and don't hesitate to seek support from healthcare professionals as you navigate your path to recovery.

We hope this cookbook has provided you with the tools and inspiration to make every meal a positive experience. From the first week of soft foods to the final stages of incorporating a variety of textures and flavors, you have the power to create a balanced and enjoyable diet that supports your well-being.

Thank you for allowing us to be part of your journey. Here's to your continued healing, comfort, and culinary adventures!

Made in the USA
Monee, IL
15 November 2024

70200211R00105